Dietary Treatment of Epilepsy

Dietary Treatment of Epilepsy

Practical Implementation of Ketogenic Therapy

Edited by

Elizabeth Neal, RD PhD

Research Dietitian, Matthew's Friends Charity and Clinics
Honorary Research Associate, UCL-Institute of Child Health

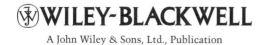
WILEY-BLACKWELL

A John Wiley & Sons, Ltd., Publication

Registered Office
John Wiley & Sons, Ltd, The Atrium, Southern Gate, Chichester, West Sussex, PO19 8SQ, UK

Editorial Offices
9600 Garsington Road, Oxford, OX4 2DQ, UK
The Atrium, Southern Gate, Chichester, West Sussex, PO19 8SQ, UK
2121 State Avenue, Ames, Iowa 50014-8300, USA

For details of our global editorial offices, for customer services and for information about how to apply for permission to reuse the copyright material in this book please see our website at www.wiley.com/wiley-blackwell.

The therapeutic diets that are described in this book require specialist medical and dietetic supervision, and their success is dependent on a multidisciplinary approach to the patient's care. Dietary treatments must be individually prescribed and should not be initiated without the support of a dietitian and a neurologist or doctor with a special interest in epilepsy. Patients, parents or carers should not make any changes to their diet treatment without consulting an appropriate member of their diet team.

Library of Congress Cataloging-in-Publication Data

Dietary treatment of epilepsy : practical implementation of ketogenic therapy / edited by Elizabeth Neal.
    p. ; cm.
  Includes bibliographical references and index.
  ISBN 978-0-470-67041-5 (pbk. : alk. paper)
  I. Neal, Elizabeth, 1965–
  [DNLM: 1. Epilepsy–diet therapy.   2. Ketogenic Diet–methods.   WL 385]
  616.85′30654–dc23

                                        2012010604

A catalogue record for this book is available from the British Library.

Wiley also publishes its books in a variety of electronic formats. Some content that appears in print may not be available in electronic books.

Set in 10.5/12.5pt Times by SPi Publisher Services, Pondicherry, India
Printed in Singapore by Ho Printing Singapore Pte Ltd

1   2012

Contents

Contributors

Christina Bergqvist
Associate Professor of Neurology
and Pediatrics and Director of
Dietary Treatment Program for
Epilepsy, Division of Neurology/
Department of Pediatrics, Children's
Hospital of Philadelphia, University
of Pennsylvania School of Medicine,
Philadelphia, USA

Hannah Chaffe
Clinical Nurse Specialist Complex
Epilepsy, UCL-Institute of Child
Health and Great Ormond Street
Hospital for Children NHS Trust,
London, UK

Jan Chapple
Paediatric Dietitian, Yorkhill
Children's Hospital, Glasgow,
Scotland, UK

J. Helen Cross
Professor, The Prince of Wales's
Chair of Childhood Epilepsy,
Neurosciences Unit, UCL-Institute
of Child Health and Great Ormond
Street Hospital for Children, London,
and National Centre for Young
Epilepsy, Lingfield, UK

Nicole Dos Santos
Paediatric Dietitian, St George's
Hospital, London, UK

Tuscha Du Toit
Specialist Dietitian, Pretoria,
South Africa

Georgiana Fitzsimmons
Paediatric Dietitian, UCL-Institute
of Child Health and Great Ormond
Street Hospital for Children NHS
Trust, London, UK

Adam L. Hartman
Assistant Professor of Neurology and
Paediatrics, Johns Hopkins Hospital,
Baltimore, USA

Hoon-Chul Kang
Associate Professor, Division of
Pediatric Neurology, Severance
Children's Hospital and Department
of Pediatrics, Yonsei University
College of Medicine, Seoul, Korea

Heung Dong Kim
Professor, Division of Pediatric
Neurology, Department of Pediatrics,
Severance Children's Hospital and
Epilepsy Research Institute, Yonsei
University College of Medicine,
Seoul, Korea

Joerg Klepper
Professor of Paediatric Neurology,
Childrens' Hospital Aschaffenburg,
Germany

Eric H. Kossoff
Associate Professor of Neurology
and Pediatrics and Medical Director
of Ketogenic Diet Center, Johns
Hopkins Hospital, Baltimore, USA

Bridget Lambert
Senior Clinical Nutritionist, Vitaflo
International Ltd, Liverpool, UK;
formerly Paediatric Dietitian, John
Radcliffe Hospital, Oxford, UK

Mary-Anne Leung
Paediatric Dietitian, Evelina
Children's Hospital, London, UK

Gwyneth Magrath
Paediatric Dietitian, Matthew's
Friends Charity and Clinics,
Lingfield, UK; formerly Paediatric
Dietitian, Birmingham Children's
Hospital, UK

Janak Nathan
Paediatric Neurologist, Shushrusha
Hospital, Mumbai, India

Elizabeth Neal
Research Dietitian, Matthew's
Friends Charity and Clinics,
Lingfield, UK and Honorary
Research Associate, Neurosciences
Unit, UCL-Institute of Child Health,
London, UK

Heidi H. Pfeifer
Pediatric Dietitian, Massachusetts
General Hospital, Boston, USA

Tara Randall
Paediatric Dietitian, Evelina
Children's Hospital, London, UK

Jong M. Rho
Professor of Paediatrics and Clinical
Neurosciences, Dr Robert Haslam
Chair in Child Neurology, University
of Calgary Faculty of Medicine and
Alberta Children's Hospital, Calgary,
Alberta, Canada

Emma Williams
Founder/CEO, Matthew's Friends
Global Charity and Director,
Matthew's Friends Clinics,
Lingfield, UK

Ruth E. Williams
Paediatric Neurologist, Evelina
Children's Hospital, London, UK

Susan Wood
Dietitian, Matthew's Friends Charity
and Clinics, Lingfield, UK

Note to readers

The therapeutic diets that are described in this book require specialist medical
and dietetic supervision, and their success is dependent on a multidisciplinary
approach to the patient's care. Dietary treatments must be individually prescribed and should not be initiated without the support of a dietitian and a
neurologist or doctor with a special interest in epilepsy. Patients, parents or
carers should not make any changes to their diet treatment without consulting
an appropriate member of their diet team.

Foreword

It gives me great pleasure to write a foreword for *Dietary Treatment of Epilepsy: Practical Implementation of Ketogenic Therapy*. This is a comprehensive book which includes much more than its title may suggest. The book fulfils two functions: it gives extensive and current evidence for the efficacy of the ketogenic regimen and also provides the know-how for healthcare professionals to safely implement and manage the diet. There is an impressive list of international contributors who are expert in their fields and the whole has been skilfully assembled by the editor so that it has a uniform style, a logical progression and is easy to read.

The book is divided into three sections. Section 1 reviews the science behind ketogenic therapies. The ketogenic diet has been slow to be accepted by healthcare professionals, particularly in the modern era of "miracle" and "celebrity" diets. Although it is not known exactly how the ketogenic diet works, the biochemistry of several possible mechanisms is explained, referring the reader to more detailed texts where appropriate. Sufficient evidence on the efficacy of diets is presented from renowned peer reviewed literature to satisfy and convince even the most sceptical.

The second section is perhaps the heart of the book as it covers in detail the practical aspects of ketogenic regimens. Every aspect of initiation, monitoring, nutritional adequacy, problems and discontinuation of the different diets is dealt with. A unique and insightful chapter is written by a parent; this should be essential reading for all who deal with children with epilepsy.

Section 3 extends the scope of the book by reviewing the use of ketogenic regimens in countries other than western economies; since 80% of people with epilepsy live in low or middle income countries this is relevant to a wide audience. The section continues by discussing the use of ketogenic diets in infants, in adults and in conditions other than epilepsy.

This book is not only for experienced dietitians (who will certainly learn from the wealth of experience of the contributors) but for other healthcare professionals including doctors, nurses, pharmacists, biochemists and anyone involved in the care of adults and children in the hospital or in the community. I am sure that this is the first of many editions of this book and that *Dietary Treatment of Epilepsy* will be the reference book on the subject for the foreseeable future.

Margaret Lawson MSc, PhD, FBDA
Senior Research Fellow, Institute of Child Health,
University College London.

A personal note

It's impossible to put into words what it feels like when you first witness your baby having a seizure – quite simply you think they are going to die. On that fateful evening I remember holding Matthew praying that he wouldn't be taken away from me as I waited for the ambulance to arrive. Little did I know that my life had just changed forever and although Matthew obviously didn't die, everything for his 'normal' future just had. My realization of that fact was going to be a long, painful and drawn-out process, as year by year I was going to witness Matthew have thousands upon thousands of seizures and more of my boy being taken away from me. It got to the stage where, once again, I would be holding him waiting for the ambulance to arrive, only this time I would be praying that he *would* die as I couldn't bear to watch his little body go through any more or listen to his screams as yet another seizure took hold of him.

I never knew about complex epilepsy. Like most of the population, I thought people with epilepsy just took medication and then they didn't have seizures any more. How naive of me. I was giving Matthew medication after medication and nothing was working. The doctor would come out with the following favourite phrases: 'just put the dose up further', 'we will add in another one' and 'we will get the right one eventually' – the 'right' medication never did turn up and every time hopes were raised and dashed and Matthew's personality had changed. His behaviour became very difficult to manage, and depending on the type of medication he was taking, at times violent and sleep-disturbed. Some of the drug 'treatments' even made the seizures worse, so you start looking for answers yourself and that is when I found the ketogenic diet.

The ketogenic diet offers something else; it offers another hope and sometimes a little hope is all we have left. When I first enquired about the ketogenic diet I was told that it was 'rubbish', that it 'didn't work' and that it was 'unpalatable and disgusting'. I believed the doctor that told me this and I rue the day that I did. Six years of asking for the diet and being refused it, until eventually when there was nothing left to try, Matthew was allowed to go on the ketogenic diet, thanks to the clinical trial that was being held at UCL-Institute of Child Health and Great Ormond Street Hospital. Within 2 weeks Matthew's seizures had reduced by 90%, he was bright, happy and relaxed and just a totally different boy; within 8 months of starting the diet he was off all medication and I got what was left of my son back. As for the diet, it wasn't disgusting, it wasn't difficult and it wasn't unpalatable. I did have to be organized and it did take up a little extra time, but once I got used to it and got myself into a routine we were away. It felt *so good* to be doing something positive in the treatment of Matthew instead of just giving him pills that made him worse. Matthew was enjoying his food as he had always done and our family life as a whole was completely different. We actually had a life and I had the chance to enjoy time with my daughter Alice.

Matthew's story is now quite well known in the ketogenic world thanks to the charity I set up in his honour. I knew that other people would be going through the same heartache that I had been through and I wanted to make sure that the correct information was available for families as well as support for them, hence Matthew's Friends was born. No one wanted to be his friend when he was younger, his epilepsy was just too frightening, but today he has friends all over the world.

To see the diet now growing in popularity, to see more children benefiting and now adults too, I am delighted to be writing for this book which will hopefully help other medical professionals to work with these diets, so giving patients a better chance at a good quality of life. For some of them it will provide the ultimate miracle of complete seizure freedom for the rest of their lives. These diets should not be the last resort.

Even today I attend seminars where I hear professionals say that ketogenic dietary therapy is difficult to do and requires a 'complete lifestyle change for the family'. Although I hasten to add this is not true, it always makes me smile because what they need to realize is that we have already been through the biggest lifestyle change you could ever imagine by living with uncontrolled complex epilepsy and all the struggles that entails. Changing a diet around is nothing compared to that. My lifestyle completely changed after that first seizure. We need to remind the families of just how far they have come and encourage them, not frighten them.

2012 now sees Matthew enter his 18th year and we are looking forward to celebrating a birthday that we never thought he would make. Matthew has been off the diet for nearly 5 years and the good effects are still with us. Matthew is a bright, happy and totally chilled-out young man with a great quality of life. He and his sister have an exceptional relationship and they are both my proudest achievement. When Matthew smiles at me every morning then I know everything is right in my world.

I could not finish this without thanking Professor Helen Cross, Dr Elizabeth Neal and Hannah Chaffe, the team at Great Ormond Street that looked after Matthew and I through his ketogenic diet treatment. A special word has to go to Matthew's dietitian, Elizabeth Neal; her kindness, understanding and support was incredible and we all worked together to make Matthew as well as he could be. I can never thank her enough and neither can Matthew. Thank you also to all the professionals that work or want to work in this field. We cannot do it without you and by choosing to work in ketogenic dietary therapy you are going to be making a huge difference to families that have already had hopes dashed and probably already been to hell and back. My promise to you is that the Matthew's Friends charity will continue to support you and the families as much as we can.

Emma Williams
Founder/CEO Matthew's Friends Global Charity,
Director Matthew's Friends Clinics

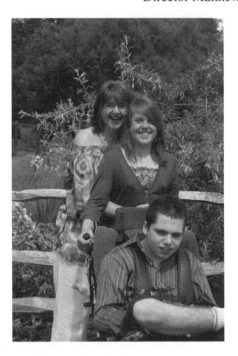

Emma, Alice (aged 15) and Matthew (aged 17)

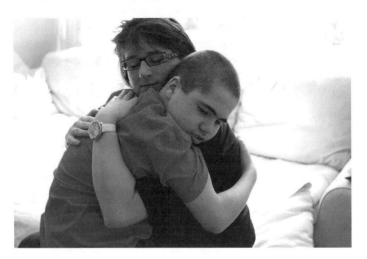

Emma and Matthew

Section 1

Introduction and Overview

Chapter 1

Introduction to the ketogenic diet and other dietary treatments

Elizabeth Neal

Matthew's Friends Charity and Clinics, Lingfield, UK

Historical overview

The idea that inclusion or abstinence from certain foods could have benefits for those with seizures has origins that far precede our current era of scientific research. A dietary approach to the treatment of epilepsy can be traced back to the 5th century BC, when Hippocrates described a man whose seizures were cured by abstaining from all food and drink. Guelpa and Marie (1911) are accredited with writing the first scientific account of the benefits of fasting in epilepsy. In 1921 Geyelin also reported the successful use of fasting, with 20 of 26 fasted patients showing improved seizure control, two remaining seizure-free for over a year. The arbitrary length of fasting was 20 days, although only four had seizures after the tenth day without food (Geyelin, 1921). Geyelin was inspired by the work of Conklin, an osteopath who believed that epilepsy was caused by the release of a toxin from the Peyer's patches of the intestine which was taken up by the lymphatic system and periodically released into the blood, triggering seizures. Conklin therefore advocated complete gut rest and starved his patients for up to 25 days. He reported a 90 % success rate in children under the age of 10 years, decreasing to 50 % in those aged 25–40 years; success was more limited in the older adults (Conklin, 1922). These observations sparked considerable clinical and research interest, and linked with ongoing studies examining ketoacidosis and the disturbance in glucose metabolism that occurs in diabetes.

During starvation, the body passes through various phases of metabolic adaptation to spare muscle protein breakdown and draw on the energy reserves of body fat. Skeletal muscle and other tissues progressively switch energy source from glucose to free fatty acids generated from triglyceride breakdown. There is increased oxidation of fatty acids in the liver, with increased production of the water-soluble ketone bodies acetoacetate and β-hydroxybutyrate. Ketone bodies

Dietary Treatment of Epilepsy: Practical Implementation of Ketogenic Therapy,
First Edition. Edited by Elizabeth Neal.

can be used as an alternative fuel by many tissues, most notably the brain, as unlike fatty acids they are able to pass across the blood–brain barrier. Blood ketone-body levels will continue to increase during the first 3 weeks of starvation during which the brain adapts to them as its primary energy source. (See Chapter 5 for further detail on biochemical changes and their connection with our current understanding of how dietary treatments may work.)

Prolonged starvation as a means to treat epilepsy had obvious practical limitations, and it was first suggested by Wilder (1921a) that a diet very high in fat and low in carbohydrate might mimic the benefits of fasting by causing a similar ketotic effect. He tried this proposed 'ketogenic diet' (KD) on three of his patients at the Mayo Clinic and reported significant seizure control (Wilder, 1921b). Peterman, a fellow worker at the clinic, reported further successful results in children treated with this KD (Peterman, 1924). Talbot and his co-workers introduced the idea of a preliminary fast before commencing the diet, with a gradual build-up of dietary fat over the following few days. His clear instructions on how to calculate the diet form the basis of the classical KD calculations used widely today (Talbot et al., 1927; Talbot, 1930; see Chapter 8).

Other early studies also reported the wide use and success of the KD (Helmholz, 1927; McQuarrie and Keith, 1927; Lennox, 1928; Wilkins, 1937). The discovery of new anticonvulsant drugs at the end of the 1930s distracted clinical and research interest from diet and towards medications, the latter perceived to be both simpler and more palatable to use. Increasing realization that not all seizures respond to drugs and concerns about medication side effects and the possible ramifications of prolonged intractable seizures, especially in the context of childhood development, have renewed interest in dietary treatments. The past few decades have seen a steady proliferation of published research, accompanied by a broadening of clinical application extending beyond the traditional classical form of KD. While this is still used extensively today, alternative types of KD therapy have allowed a more flexible approach to dietary treatments for epilepsy.

The classical and medium-chain triglyceride KD

Early studies in children by Wilder, Peterman and Talbot used a diet of 1 g protein per kilogram body weight, with 10–15 g carbohydrate daily, the remaining energy supply being from fat. Fat was primarily animal based, in the form of butter, lard and cream. The term 'ketogenic ratio' was used to describe the ratio of ketone-producing foods in the diet (fat) to foods that reduced ketone production (carbohydrate and protein). Seizure control was found to be optimal with a ratio of 3 or more. This led to the terminology of a 3 : 1 KD (87 % of total dietary energy derived from fat) or 4 : 1 KD (90 % of total dietary energy derived from fat). This is the basis of the classical KD used today. Carbohydrate intake is very limited: bread, cereals, pasta or rice are generally not allowed, the main carbohydrate sources being controlled portions of vegetables or fruit at each meal. Protein is

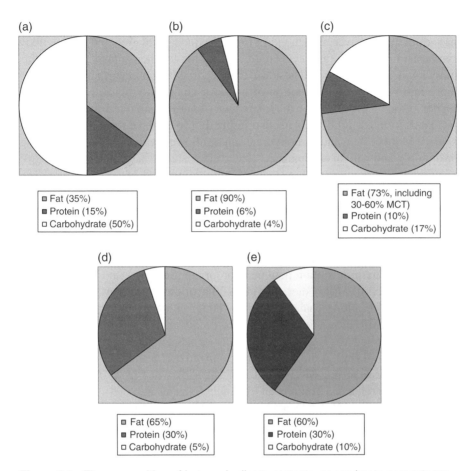

(a)

□ Fat (35%)
■ Protein (15%)
□ Carbohydrate (50%)

(b)

□ Fat (90%)
■ Protein (6%)
□ Carbohydrate (4%)

(c)

□ Fat (73%, including
   30-60% MCT)
■ Protein (10%)
□ Carbohydrate (17%)

(d)

□ Fat (65%)
■ Protein (30%)
□ Carbohydrate (5%)

(e)

□ Fat (60%)
■ Protein (30%)
□ Carbohydrate (10%)

Figure 1.1   The composition of ketogenic diet treatments: approximate percentages of dietary energy from fat, protein and carbohydrate. (a) Recommended UK diet; (b) classical 4 : 1 ratio ketogenic diet; (c) MCT ketogenic diet; (d) modified Atkins diet (at 1 : 1 ketogenic ratio); (e) low glycaemic index treatment.

kept to a minimum to meet requirements: a source can be included at each meal, such as meat, fish, egg or cheese, but protein foods that contain additional sources of carbohydrate are generally avoided. The macronutrient composition of this type of diet is substantially different from an average UK diet (Figure 1.1).

A modification of the classical KD was proposed in 1971, using medium-chain triglyceride (MCT) as an alternative fat source (Huttenlocher et al., 1971). The main constituents of MCT are the medium-chain octanoic and decanoic fatty acids, which are absorbed more efficiently than their long-chain counterparts, and which are carried to the liver in portal blood bound to albumin. This is in contrast to long-chain fatty acids, which are incorporated into chylomicrons and transported via the thoracic duct through the lymph system, exiting into the circulation at the left subclavian vein from where they are carried via peripheral tissues to the liver. After hepatic tissue uptake, medium-chain fatty acids can pass directly into liver mitochondria for subsequent oxidation and ketone body synthesis. Long-chain fatty acids require carnitine for their transport across this mitochondrial membrane. These differences in MCT metabolism facilitate a more rapid and greater oxidation of medium-chain fatty acids, resulting in a higher ketone yield per kilocalorie of dietary energy than that from long-chain fat. Therefore less total fat is needed in the diet to achieve the desired level of ketosis. More protein and carbohydrate can be allowed with the aim of improving palatability and patient acceptance.

Huttenlocher went on to show that a KD providing 60 % of total dietary energy from MCT was as effective as a 3 : 1 classical diet in producing ketosis and controlling seizures in 12 children with epilepsy (Huttenlocher, 1976). This amount of ingested MCT, particularly if introduced too quickly, can cause gastrointestinal side effects, primarily diarrhoea and abdominal discomfort. Although these can be ameliorated with dietary adjustment, in some individuals a more moderate prescription may be appropriate. Schwartz and her colleagues suggested a modified MCT diet, providing 30 % of dietary energy from MCT and an extra 30 % from long-chain fats such as butter or cream; this has been termed the John Radcliffe diet. They also reported no difference between the classical, MCT and modified MCT KDs in controlling seizures in a non-randomized study (Schwartz et al., 1989). A more recent randomized trial by our group also showed neither the classical nor MCT KD to be superior when assessing efficacy or tolerability after 3, 6 or 12 months of treatment (Neal et al., 2009). Further details on the classical and MCT KD can be found in Chapters 8 and 9.

Alternative KD therapies

In the last decade two other types of KD therapy have been used with success. The modified Atkins diet (MAD) was first used in 2002 for two children at the Johns Hopkins Hospital in Baltimore, USA. One child was waiting for a scheduled admission to start the classical KD; another had discontinued classical KD a year before. Seizures were successfully controlled with the MAD in both cases (Kossoff et al., 2003). This diet restricts carbohydrates, encourages high-fat foods, but does not limit or measure protein or total calories. The principles are based on the popular weight loss diet first described by Dr Robert C. Atkins in 1972 (Atkins, 1972), with the primary outcome goal of weight loss replaced by one of seizure control. Carbohydrate is usually restricted to 10–20 g per day and review of dietary records shows that the approximate ratio of fat to carbohydrate and protein is 1 : 1 compared with 3 : 1 or 4 : 1 with the classical KD. There is a growing body of scientific publications reporting successful use of the MAD.

An alternative diet, the low glycaemic index treatment (LGIT), was first described in 2005 (Pfeifer and Thiele, 2005). This diet restricts carbohydrates to 40–60 g per day but only allows those with a glycaemic index of less than 50, the aim being to minimize increases in blood glucose. Food is not weighed but based on portion sizes. Protein, fat and calorie intake is loosely monitored, albeit considerably less strictly than on traditional KDs. Unlike the MAD, a high-fat intake is not actively encouraged.

Figure 1.1 illustrates the differences in dietary composition of these alternative dietary treatments as compared with traditional KDs. Because of the flexible nature of the MAD and LGIT, the percentages of energy from the different macronutrients may vary between individual diets; the figures chosen give the reader some idea of how an average diet might look. Further details on the MAD and LGIT can be found in Chapters 10 and 11.

Other non-KD treatments

There have been suggestions that food intolerance could be linked to epilepsy in the literature, although these are mostly anecdotal and uncontrolled reports. A 1968 review of 26 studies examining a relationship between epilepsy and allergies concluded that pollen, dust and moulds were the main culprits (Fein and Kamin, 1968). In a study examining the role of oligoantigenic diets in 63 children with epilepsy, 45 of whom had associated headaches, abdominal symptoms or hyperkinetic behaviour, 37 had improved seizures on an elimination diet (Egger et al., 1989). However, the 18 children with epilepsy alone showed no improvement. A further study of the same elimination diet failed to demonstrate any benefit in nine children with epilepsy (Van Someren et al., 1990). Although it is possible that allergic reactions could trigger seizures in susceptible patients, the present evidence does not support the use of elimination diets in epilepsy treatment and further detail on this type of dietary therapy is not included in this book.

Application and availability of KD therapy

The classical and MCT KDs are primarily used in children, although studies have demonstrated benefit in infants (Nordli et al., 2001; Hong et al., 2010), adolescents (Mady et al., 2003) and adults (Sirven et al., 1999); the MAD has also been demonstrated effective in treating adults (Kossoff et al., 2008a). The flexible protocols employed in both the MAD and LGIT are clearly useful for adolescents and adults with epilepsy who may prefer a less rigid dietary treatment, but they can also be used with success as an alternative for children. Although most of this book will refer to children, a separate chapter on adults is also included. As well as being successfully used to treat epilepsy in all age groups, the KD is an important treatment for two metabolic disorders, glucose transporter (GLUT)-1 deficiency and pyruvate dehydrogenase deficiency (see Chapter 27).

Worldwide use of the KD has increased dramatically since the early 1990s. Although the greatest number of centres offering this treatment are in the USA, a survey reported KD programmes in 41 other countries, 16 of which had multiple centres (Kossoff and McGrogan, 2005). Most geographic regions were represented, with the exception of the majority of Africa and Central America. Most of the larger centres in the USA used a classical KD protocol at the time of this survey, but European and worldwide KD practice was more varied, with both classical and MCT diets being employed. Both protocols are used within the UK; a postal survey of 280 British Dietetic Association Paediatric Group members in 2000 found 22 centres were using the KD, 13 the classical and nine the MCT (Magrath et al., 2000). The survey was repeated in 2007 and although use of the KD had risen by 50 %, numbers were still small as this only represented an increase of 51 patients (Lord and Magrath, 2010). At the time of this survey, no dietitians reported using MAD or LGIT. Similar to reports from other European centres (Kossoff and McGrogan, 2005), a lack of funding resources and dietetic time was identified as the main barrier to greater use of dietary treatments. Since these studies were published, practice has changed considerably, with many more centres in the UK and around the world now using the MAD, and a smaller but growing number the LGIT. Using MAD as a dietary treatment for epilepsy in developing countries is also being explored (Kossoff et al., 2008b). Neurologists are becoming more aware of dietary therapies, but many continue to reserve its use until a child has failed a number of anticonvulsants.

The successful use of more relaxed KD therapies is leading the way towards a flexible, rather than rigid, approach to dietary treatment of epilepsy; this may include components of the various protocols drawn together to provide a treatment individually tailored to specific dietary and lifestyle requirements. A clear understanding of how the different types of diet are calculated and implemented is essential before they can be adapted in such a way and this book aims to provide the information to help foster this understanding. The inclusion of guidance on when to use KD therapy, how to initiate, calculate, fine-tune, monitor and discontinue treatments, the potential side effects, use in infants and adults as well as children, and practical advice from both parent and dietitian, will provide readers with a comprehensive and practical training on all aspects of implementation.

References

Atkins, R.C. (1972) *Dr. Atkins' Diet Revolution*. Bantam Books: New York.

Conklin, H.W. (1922) Cause and treatment of epilepsy. *J Am Osteopath Assoc* **26**, 11–14.

Egger, J., Carter, C.M., Soothill, J.F. and Wilson, J. (1989) Oligoantigenic diet treatment of children with epilepsy and migraine. *J Pediatr* **114**, 51–58.

Fein, B.T. and Kamin, P.B. (1968) Allergy, convulsive disorders and epilepsy. *Ann Allergy* **26**, 241–247.

Geyelin, H.R. (1921) Fasting as a method for treating epilepsy. *Medical Record* **99**, 1037–1039.

Guelpa, G. and Marie, A. (1911) La lutte contre l'epilepsie par la desintoxication et par la reducation alimentaire. *Revue de Therapie Medico-Chirurgicale* **78**, 8–13.

Helmholz, H.F. (1927) The treatment of epilepsy in childhood: five years' experience with the ketogenic diet. *JAMA* **88**, 2028–2032.

Hong, A.M., Hamdy, R.F., Turner, Z. and Kossoff, E.H. (2010) Infantile spasms treated with the ketogenic diet: prospective single-center experience in 104 consecutive infants. *Epilepsia* **51**, 1403–1407.

Huttenlocher, P.R. (1976) Ketonaemia and seizures: metabolic and anticonvulsant effects of two ketogenic diets in childhood epilepsy. *Pediatr Res* **10**, 536–540.

Huttenlocher, P.R., Wilbourne, A.J. and Sigmore, J.M. (1971) Medium chain triglycerides as a therapy for intractable childhood epilepsy. *Neurology* **21**, 1097–1103.

Kossoff, E.H. and McGrogan, J.R. (2005) Worldwide use of the ketogenic diet. *Epilepsia* **46**, 280–289.

Kossoff, E.H., Krauss, G.L., McGrogan, J.R. and Freeman, J.M. (2003) Efficacy of the Atkins Diet as therapy for intractable epilepsy. *Neurology* **61**, 1789–1791.

Kossoff, E.H., Rowley, H., Sinha, S.R. and Vining, E.P.G. (2008a) A prospective study of the modified Atkins diet for intractable epilepsy in adults. *Epilepsia* **49**, 316–319.

Kossoff, E.H., Dorward, J.L., Molinero, M.R. and Holden, K.R. (2008b) The Modified Atkins Diet: a potential treatment for developing countries. *Epilepsia* **49**, 1646–1647.

Lennox, W.G. (1928) Ketogenic diet in the treatment of epilepsy. *N Engl J Med* **199**, 74–75.

Lord, K. and Magrath, G. (2010) Use of the ketogenic diet and dietary practices in the UK. *J Hum Nutr Diet* **23**, 126–132.

McQuarrie, I. and Keith, H.M. (1927) Epilepsy in children. Relationship of variations in the degree of ketonuria to occurrence of convulsions in epileptic children on ketogenic diets. *Am J Dis Child* **34**, 1013–1029.

Mady, M.A., Kossoff, E.H., McGregor, A.L., Wheless, J.W., Pyzik, P.L. and Freeman, J.M. (2003) The ketogenic diet: adolescents can do it, too. *Epilepsia* **44**, 847–851.

Magrath, G., MacDonald, A. and Whitehouse, W. (2000) Dietary practices and use of the ketogenic diet in the UK. *Seizure* **9**, 128–130.

Neal, E.G., Chaffe, H.M., Schwartz, R. et al. (2009) A randomised trial of classical and medium-chain triglyceride ketogenic diets in the treatment of childhood epilepsy. *Epilepsia* **50**, 1109–1117.

Nordli, D.R., Kuroda, M.M., Carroll, J. et al. (2001) Experience with the ketogenic diet in infants. *Pediatrics* **108**, 129–133.

Peterman, M.G. (1924) The ketogenic diet in the treatment of epilepsy: a preliminary report. *Am J Dis Child* **28**, 28–33.

Pfeifer, H.H. and Thiele, E.A. (2005) Low glycemic-index treatment: a liberalized ketogenic diet for treatment of intractable epilepsy. *Neurology* **65**, 1810–1812.

Schwartz, R.H., Eaton, J., Bower, B.D. and Aynsley-Green, A. (1989) Ketogenic diets in the treatment of epilepsy: short term clinical effects. *Dev Med Child Neurol* **31**, 145–151.

Sirven, J., Whedon, B., Caplan, D. et al. (1999) The ketogenic diet for intractable epilepsy in adults: preliminary results. *Epilepsia* **40**, 1721–1726.

Talbot, F.B. (1930) *Treatment of Epilepsy*. New York: Macmillian.

Talbot, F.B., Metcalf, K.M. and Moriarty, M.E. (1927) A clinical study of epileptic children treated by the ketogenic diet. *Boston Medical and Surgical Journal* **196**, 89–96.

Van Someren, V.V., Robinson, R.O., Mcardle, B. and Sturgeon, N. (1990) Restricted diets for treatment of migraine. *J Pediatr* **117**, 509–510.

Wilder, R.M. (1921a) The effects of ketonemia on the course of epilepsy. *Mayo Clinic Proc* **2**, 307.

Wilder, R.M. (1921b) High fat diets in epilepsy. *Mayo Clinic Proc* **2**, 308.

Wilkins, L. (1937) Epilepsy in childhood. III: Results with the ketogenic diet. *J Pediatr* **10**, 341–357.

Chapter 2

Epilepsy and epileptic seizures

J. Helen Cross

UCL-Institute of Child Health and Great Ormond Street Hospital for Children, London, UK

Epilepsy is a diagnosis given when an individual is prone to recurrent epileptic seizures. By definition an epileptic seizure is a change in movement or behaviour that is the direct result of a primary change in the electrical activity of the brain. Up to 1 in 20 individuals will have an epileptic seizure in their lifetime; only 1 in 200 will experience more than two seizures and therefore be given a diagnosis of epilepsy. Epilepsy is a symptom and there are many different causes; it would be more accurate to term the condition 'the epilepsies'. Moreover, there is no single diagnostic test. Diagnosis is made on the assessment of description of events by experienced physicians with support from results of investigations. Prognosis will depend on the type and cause of the epilepsy; further decisions about management and need and type of treatment will also be dependent on the underlying diagnosis and type of epilepsy.

Diagnosis

An epileptic seizure can be defined as an intermittent and stereotyped disturbance of consciousness, behaviour, emotion, motor function or sensation that on clinical grounds is believed to result from cortical neuronal discharge, determined as a change in the electrical activity of the brain. Epilepsy is defined as a condition in which unprovoked (namely not triggered by an acute condition) seizures recur, usually spontaneously. Consequently, by definition, an individual is diagnosed as having epilepsy if he or she has had at least two epileptic seizures. Diagnosis can be challenging. As there remains no diagnostic test, a diagnosis should be made by a physician with an expertise in epilepsy, in the case of children by a paediatrician, as the diagnosis will be made on the basis of description of events by an eyewitness. Events suggestive of epileptic seizures may occur as the result of a

Dietary Treatment of Epilepsy: Practical Implementation of Ketogenic Therapy,
First Edition. Edited by Elizabeth Neal.

Box 2.1   Differential diagnosis for epilepsy in children.

Syncope and related disorders
Disorders of orthostatic control: reflex syncope
Respiratory syncope
  Reflex and expiratory apnoeic syncope
  'Fainting lark'
  Upper airway obstruction
Cardiac syncope
  Arrhythmias
  Complete heart block
  Wolf–Parkinson–White syndrome
Brainstem syncope
  Tumour
  Brainstem herniation or compression
Other: anoxic epileptic seizures

Neurological
Tics
Myoclonus
Paroxysmal dystonia
Sandifer syndrome
Paroxysmal dyskinesias
Cataplexy
Benign paroxysmal vertigo/torticollis
Migraine
Alternating hemiplegia
Eye movement disorders
Overflow movements
Hyperekplexia

Behavioural/psychiatric
Daydreams
Dissociative states
Self-gratification behaviour
Hyperventilation
Panic/anxiety
Non-epileptic attack disorder
Fabricated attacks
Pseudosyncope
Stereotypies/ritualistic behaviour

Sleep disorders
Sleep myoclonus
Headbanging
Confusional arousal
REM sleep disorder/night terrors

secondary change to the electrical activity of the brain, for example the result of other causes of collapse such as syncope or heart arrhythmias. The range of differential diagnosis is particularly wide in children (Box 2.1). The misdiagnosis rate is consequently high; up to 40% of children attending a tertiary clinic for an opinion for epilepsy may subsequently prove not to have the condition.

The key investigation in the evaluation of an individual with a history of epileptic seizures is the electroencephalogram (EEG). This is carried out using a standard placement of silver electrodes on the head, with recordings taken between each of two points. An EEG should be performed in all individuals with a history of at least two epileptic seizures. Although unlikely to be diagnostic unless the individual experiences an event during the recording, specific abnormalities identified either as deviant from what is normally expected for the age of the individual, or epileptiform activity (spikes and sharp waves) may not only support the clinical diagnosis but also aid toward a diagnosis of the type of epilepsy (Figure 2.1). Magnetic resonance imaging (MRI) of the brain is likely to be performed in many individuals at diagnosis, but will only give information about a possible underlying cause rather than help toward the diagnosis of epilepsy itself. Other investigations selected thereafter, for example to exclude a metabolic cause, will depend on the overall clinical presentation and will only be performed in a select number of individuals presenting with perhaps other symptomatology.

Prevalence and incidence

Despite differing definitions of epilepsy and case ascertainment methods, there is remarkable agreement about the epidemiology of epilepsy in different populations in the developed world. Incidence rates vary between 20 and 55 per 100 000 per year whereas the prevalence for active epilepsy (those on medication or a history of a seizure in the last 5 years) is in the range of 4–10 per 1000. The incidence of epilepsy is highest at the extremes of life, with an incidence in those under the age of 2 years of 60–80 per 100 000. There are significant differences between cumulative incidence and prevalence of epilepsy, indicating that the majority of patients who develop epilepsy do not suffer from a chronic disorder. Incidence and prevalence are higher in developing as opposed to developed countries, with higher rates usually found in rural as opposed to urban communities.

Epileptic seizure and syndrome diagnosis

At diagnosis, it is important to determine not only whether the individual has epilepsy but also thereafter the seizure types, and ultimately where possible to diagnose the electroclinical syndrome. Epileptic seizures are broadly defined as generalized or focal in onset. A generalized seizure is defined as one that originates, and rapidly engages, bilaterally distributed networks – namely that wide areas of the cerebral cortex on both sides of the brain are involved rapidly from the onset. There are different manifestations of generalized seizures (Box 2.2) dependent on the relative movements and degree of musculature involved. A focal seizure (also termed partial seizure) is one that originates

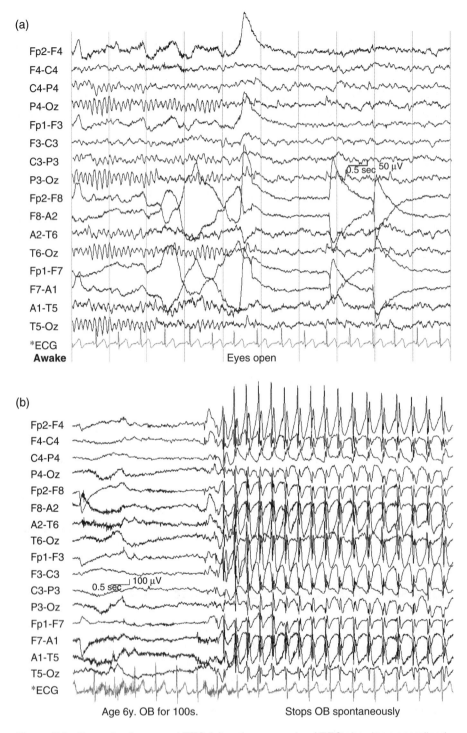

Figure 2.1 Example of a normal EEG (a) and an example of EEG showing generalized spike wave activity seen in childhood absence epilepsy (b).

Box 2.2   Classification of seizure types.

Generalized seizures
General tonic–clonic
Absence
  Typical
  Atypical
  Absence with special features
    Myoclonic absence
    Absence with eyelid myoclonia
Myoclonic
  Myoclonic
  Myoclonic atonic
  Myoclonic tonic
Tonic
Atonic

Focal seizures

Epileptic spasms

within a single network within one hemisphere, which is then further described according to severity (loss of consciousness, evolution to convulsive seizure) and likely site of origin. The latter will be surmised from the clinical presentation of the seizure, for example epigastric warning, and subsequent automatisms in individuals with seizures likely to be of temporal lobe origin. A third seizure type, epileptic spasms, is now included separately within the classification as it has not been resolved whether these are focal or generalized in origin.

On determining the likely seizure type, or types, with which an individual has presented, it is important thereafter to try to determine the likely epilepsy syndrome. An epilepsy syndrome is defined as a group of clinical entities that are reliably identified by a cluster of electroclinical characteristics, namely evidence from the clinical seizure type and EEG. Patients whose epilepsy does not fit the criteria for a specific syndrome can be described with respect to a variety of clinically relevant factors, and may thereafter be also described by the underlying cause (Box 2.3). The syndromes currently described are age related, and may have different causes. The diagnosis of the likely syndrome will subsequently guide the best course of management.

There are of course many underlying causes of epilepsy that may manifest as differing epilepsy syndromes. These have been tentatively classified as genetic (where the epilepsy is the direct result of a known or inferred genetic defect(s) and seizures are the core symptom of the disorder), structural–metabolic (where there is a distinct structural or metabolic condition present) or unknown (because there remain a number of epilepsies with no known underlying cause). There is no question that advances in genetics and neuroimaging have greatly enhanced our understanding of the underlying causes of the epilepsies. Cortical malformations have been now determined to be a major cause of drug-resistant epilepsy. Further,

Box 2.3   Epilepsy syndromes.

Age 0–12 months
Benign familial neonatal convulsions
Benign idiopathic neonatal convulsions
Benign familial partial epilepsy of infancy
Early infantile epileptic encephalopathy (Ohtahara)
Early myoclonic encephalopathy
West syndrome
Dravet syndrome
Lesional focal epilepsy
Migrating partial seizures of infancy

Age 1–5 years
Panyiotopolous syndrome
Myoclonic astatic epilepsy
Lennox–Gastaut syndrome
Landau–Kleffner syndrome
Continuous spike wave of slow sleep

Age 5–10 years
Benign epilepsy with centrotemporal spikes
Late onset childhood occipital epilepsy (Gastaut type)
Autosomal dominant nocturnal frontal lobe epilepsy
Childhood absence epilepsy
Myoclonic absence epilepsy

Age over 10 years
Juvenile absence epilepsy
Juvenile myoclonic epilepsy
Progressive myoclonic epilepsies

increasingly specific gene defects coding for sodium and potassium channels have also been determined as major causes of some of the well-defined syndromes with onset in early childhood, for example sodium channel (*SCN1A*) mutations in Dravet syndrome. Specific metabolic defects have also been discovered to be a cause of paroxysmal movement disorders and epilepsy, which may have specific implications for treatment, for example glucose transporter defects.

Treatment: what and why

Once a diagnosis of epilepsy has been made, discussion is then undertaken about whether treatment is warranted, and indeed which treatment. In some circumstances, such as benign epilepsy with centrotemporal spikes, if seizures are rare a family may decide not to treat. However, the risks of the epilepsy have to be taken into consideration when any such decision is made, and in most this warrants medication. Risks include those of the seizures themselves, either through injury or accidents, or impact on learning, and in those with continuing convulsive seizures there is the risk of sudden unexplained death in epilepsy, affecting around 1 in 200.

Antiepileptic drugs (AEDs) are the first-line treatment; these medications suppress the tendency to seizures rather than treat any underlying cause. The choice of AED will depend on the epilepsy diagnosis, particularly the likely syndrome diagnosis, as well as the individual. All AEDs have reported side effects (see Chapter 3) and these possibilities have to be discussed along with the risk of recurring seizures. General principles of treatment include only ever making one change at a time, careful evaluation of any response, and trying to minimize anticonvulsant load to one drug where possible. There is no evidence to suggest that a combination of more than two drugs leads to any better control than a single drug, and toxicity is more likely to occur where multiple drugs are used together. Minimizing drug load is therefore imperative. How long treatment is required will also depend on the type of epilepsy, specifically the likelihood of spontaneous remission. Traditionally, a seizure-free period of 2 years has been suggested before considering withdrawal of medication, but the type of epilepsy and possible likelihood of remission should be carefully evaluated prior to any decision. If seizures are not controlled with up to two AEDs, consideration should be given to other options (see Chapter 3).

Prognosis

The overall prognosis for an individual with epilepsy will be related to the underlying epilepsy syndrome, as well as the underlying cause. There are a group of epilepsies presenting in childhood for which the prognosis for seizure control and remission from seizures remains extremely good. Other epilepsies presenting later (e.g. juvenile myoclonic epilepsy) may have a good prognosis for seizure control with medication, but the medication is likely to be required long term. Two-thirds of individuals with epilepsy will either become seizure-free on AEDs or enter spontaneous remission. However, one-third continues to have seizures despite appropriate use of medication. There also remains a high rate of cognitive and behavioural disorder, particularly amongst children with very early onset epilepsy. The term 'epileptic encephalopathy' has been incorporated into recent proposals for the classification of the epilepsies. Although previously a term generated to describe a certain number of early-onset epilepsy syndromes with particularly poor prognosis for cognitive development, it is now defined as a concept, in the most recent International League Against Epilepsy (ILAE) proposal, that could be applied to any epilepsy at any age. It is defined as the notion that the epileptic activity itself is contributing to cognitive and behavioural impairments beyond that expected from the underlying pathology alone (e.g. cortical malformation) and that these can worsen over time. Inevitably in each individual differing contributions may be made to any neurodevelopmental impairment from epilepsy-related factors (seizures, ongoing epileptic activity), underlying cause and the medication, and all must be weighed up carefully when decisions about treatment are being made.

Overall, quality of life in individuals with epilepsy has been found to be most significantly related to seizure control, although other life factors may contribute. However, perception of quality of life will depend on whose perspective it is viewed from. Parents' ability to manage the epilepsy and adjust psychologically will exert the most influence on their child's quality of life and minimize the risks of the psychosocial burden of the epilepsy on their child.

Summary

Epilepsy is a clinical diagnosis made when an individual has had at least two epileptic seizures. Accuracy of diagnosis of seizure type, and epilepsy syndrome, is imperative for appropriate management in the long term. Prognosis for many is good, with a high chance of seizure control and/or remission. However, there a high rate of cognitive and behavioural difficulty, especially in those with early-onset and continuing seizures. For each individual, ongoing discussion as to optimal management is required to optimize quality of life.

Further reading

Arzimanoglou, A., Guerrini, R. and Aicardi, J. (2004) *Aicardi's Epilepsy in Children*, 3rd edn. Philadelphia: Lippincott Williams & Wilkins.

Berg, A.T., Berkovic, S.F., Buchhalter, J. et al. (2010) Revised terminology and concepts for organization of seizures and epilepsies: report of the ILAE Commission on Classification and Terminology, 2005–2009. *Epilepsia* **51**, 676–685.

Cross, J.H. (2009) Pitfalls in the diagnosis and differential diagnosis of epilepsy. *Paediatr Child Health* **19**, 199–202.

Roger, J., Bureau, M., Dravet, C., Genton, P., Tassinari, C.A. and Wolf, P. (eds) (2005) *Epileptic Syndromes in Infancy, Childhood and Adolescence*, 4th edn. London: John Libbey.

Chapter 3

Treatment options in the paediatric epilepsy clinic

Ruth E. Williams

Evelina Children's Hospital, London, UK

In around 20–30% of children with epilepsy, seizures cannot be controlled easily with medication. These children may be taking two or more antiepileptic drugs (AEDs) but continue to have seizures more than once per month. Many will have experienced side effects from medication, precluding the use of sufficiently high dosage regimens to achieve seizure control. In the UK, they will have been under the care of a general paediatrician who may or may not have particular training and expertise in children's epilepsy. The UK National Institute for Health and Clinical Excellence (NICE) guidelines suggest that all such children be referred for a specialist assessment by a neurologist (NICE, 2004). The initial assessment will look at a number of issues including the underlying cause of the epilepsy and need for further diagnostic investigations (see Chapter 2), comorbidities (e.g. learning and thinking, attention and social communication skills) and their relationship with the epilepsy, and management options that will include consideration of dietary therapy. The child and family may also be introduced to other members of the multidisciplinary children's epilepsy team including an epilepsy nurse specialist. This chapter describes the management options which may be considered alongside dietary therapy.

Further trials of medication

For some children a review of the underlying cause of epilepsy and epilepsy syndrome will provide a clear path for further trials of medication. Before consideration of dietary therapy or invasive management options such as surgery, it is important that appropriate AEDs are tried in appropriate doses for an appropriate length of time. Side effects of AEDs are not uncommon (Table 3.1) and the more medications taken by a child at any one time, the

Dietary Treatment of Epilepsy: Practical Implementation of Ketogenic Therapy,
First Edition. Edited by Elizabeth Neal.

Table 3.1 Common examples of side effects of antiepileptic medication.

Type of side effect	Some examples
Predictable, mild and common at the start of treatment	Drowsiness with carbamazepine, vigabatrin
Predictable at high doses or rapid escalation	Drowsiness and nausea with ethosuximide
	Increased appetite and weight gain with valproate
	Poor appetite and weight loss with topiramate
	Rash, double vision and sleep disturbance with lamotrigine
	Tremor with valproate
	Acne and gum hypertrophy with phenytoin
	Blurred vision and unsteadiness with carbamazepine
Idiosyncratic	Hair loss, liver dysfunction and pancreatitis with valproate
	Behaviour disturbance with levetiracetam
	Bone marrow suppression with carbamazepine
Drug interactions	Increased blood levels of carbamazepine (drowsiness) with some antibiotics (e.g. erythromycin)
	Decreased effectiveness of lamotrigine when oral contraceptive pill added
Fetal toxicity (Morrow et al., 2006)	Valproate especially but not solely; more problems with polytherapy and higher doses

higher the risk of drug interactions and side effects. The impact of AEDs on thinking and learning skills, attention, sleep and behaviour cannot be underestimated. Side effects can be grouped according to their predictability and timing in relation to starting new AED treatment. Some side effects are idiosyncratic: they come unpredictably and are rare, but may be severe. Other side effects are more common, predictable and relatively mild. Other AED-related symptoms are predictable but related to high doses or rapid increases of dosage (toxicity). Some AED side effects are the result of drug interactions, for example if a child needs antibiotics for an intercurrent infection blood levels of some AEDs may be altered in a predictable way, potentially leading either to toxicity or to seizure relapse.

The place of dietary therapy

Dietary therapy for epilepsy is discussed in detail in the following chapters. For those children whose seizures have not responded to two or more medications within 1–2 years of seizure onset, and are under the care of a paediatric neurologist, dietary therapy may be considered prior to, or alongside work-up for consideration of, resective epilepsy surgery, stimulation techniques or a change of direction towards palliative care.

Epilepsy surgery

Epilepsy is a chronic condition. For perhaps the majority of children, epilepsy remains a childhood condition that does not persist into adulthood. However, for a large minority, the tendency to have seizures persists into adulthood and is expected to be lifelong; AED treatment therefore aims to control or suppress seizures but cannot cure epilepsy. A structural brain lesion can be identified in a proportion of children with epilepsy. In some, this structural abnormality can be shown to be responsible for the seizures and is amenable to resective surgery. For these children and adults, surgery represents a potential curative treatment if the entire epileptogenic zone can be removed without high risk of consequent functional impairment (e.g. hemispherectomies, lobar resections, lesionectomies). Disrupting the connections between one hemisphere of the brain and the other may prevent spread of seizure activity and clinical seizures, thus possibly modifying the disease course but considered mainly to control symptoms (e.g. functional hemispherectomy, callosotomy, subpial transection).

Deep brain stimulation and vagal nerve stimulation

Deep brain stimulation (DBS) involves the insertion of stimulation electrodes that deliver cyclical pulses of electrical current into the deep grey matter of the brain. This procedure has been helpful for a small number of adults and children but is only available in specialist surgical centres as part of research trials.

Vagal nerve stimulation (VNS) is now used widely for those adults and children not suitable for resective surgical procedures and who continue to have frequent troublesome seizures despite trials of several AEDs. The operation is usually performed as a day case, and involves placing a battery-operated device under the skin just below the left collarbone. Wires are attached to the device and these are placed around the left vagus nerve in the neck. The device delivers a pulsed electrical current that stimulates the left vagus nerve. This nerve carries fibres to and from the base of the brain through the skull. The current is switched on and adjusted using an external 'wand' and digital programming device. The current delivered and cycling times are adjusted over several months following implantation. The mechanism through which VNS works is not well understood. Seizures are seldom completely controlled and the majority of patients must continue to take regular AEDs. In some, medication can be reduced, thus reducing side effects. For some, the pattern of seizures changes so that seizures themselves become less prolonged or amenable to emergency treatment using a magnet swipe over the stimulator device to deliver a boost of current. For some individuals the recovery following a seizure is much quicker so that normal activities can be resumed. The full benefit of VNS may not be seen for 6–12 months after implantation and AEDs are seldom changed during this time.

Evaluation: is this child a candidate for surgery, DBS or VNS?

The decision to offer epilepsy surgery or stimulation to a child with epilepsy is made by a team experienced in the care of children with refractory epilepsy. The team commonly comprises paediatric and adult epileptologists/neurologists, a neuroradiologist (to interpret brain imaging including MRI, computed tomography and more specialist scans), paediatric and adult neurophysiologists (to interpret tests such as EEG and telemetry), a psychologist and/or child and adolescent psychiatrist, specialist nurses, sometimes therapists (physiotherapist, speech and language and occupational therapists as necessary) and of course the specialist paediatric epilepsy neurosurgeons. These teams are based at large neurology and neurosurgical centres and many of the investigations and tests necessary for the evaluation can only be performed in these large specialist centres. Almost all children will have undergone a period of EEG video-telemetry over several days as an inpatient, together with detailed brain MRI using special epilepsy protocols (a longer scan which may need to be performed with sedation or anaesthesia in order to provide the best-quality images). Other assessments, including motor skills, thinking and learning skills and emotional well-being, may also have been necessary. This detailed evaluation often takes time (at least months) before the most appropriate treatment course can be defined and then offered to the child and family. During the process, some children may be offered further AED trials or dietary therapy.

Palliative care

Unfortunately for a very small number of children with epilepsy, seizures cannot be controlled using any of the options above or by dietary therapy. This may be because the treatments do not work for a particular individual or because the side effects or complications are too great. In all children and adults living with epilepsy, a balance must be struck: the potential for seizure control or reduction against any drawbacks of treatment. Often there is no available curative treatment for refractory epilepsy and children's lives may be threatened or shortened as a consequence of their severe epilepsy. A proportion of the children being considered for dietary and other treatment options for refractory epilepsy have palliative care needs according to currently accepted criteria. Palliative care is defined as

> an active and total approach to care, from the point of diagnosis or recognition, embracing physical, emotional, social and spiritual elements through to death and beyond. It focuses on enhancement of quality of life for the child or young person and support for the family and includes the management of distressing symptoms, provision of short breaks and care through death and bereavement.

Complex, or continuing, care

> is a bespoke package of care beyond what is available through core and universal services. It is provided to children with high levels of complexity or intensity of nursing care needs (ACT, 2008).

All these children and families are likely to benefit from good communication between different members of the multidisciplinary and multi-agency teams (education and social agencies as well as health) supporting them, regular review and care planning. Attention to appropriate schooling, respite care at home and outside the family home and adequate and appropriate treatment and/or support for comorbidities is crucially important.

Summary

Dietary therapy has a clear place in the management of refractory epilepsy alongside a number of other therapeutic options. Children in whom treatment with two or more different AEDs has not been successful should be referred to a paediatric neurologist for further evaluation, including consideration of dietary therapy.

Acknowledgements

The children and families of the Evelina Children's Hospital Epilepsy Service.

References

ACT (2008) Together for short lives. Available at www.act.org.uk

Morrow, J., Russell, A., Guthrie, E. et al. (2006) Malformation risks of antiepileptic drugs in pregnancy: a prospective study from the UK Epilepsy and Pregnancy Register. *J Neurol Neurosurg Psychiatry* **77**, 193–198.

NICE (2004) The epilepsies: the diagnosis and management of the epilepsies in adults and children in primary and secondary care. Available at www.nice.org.uk/nicemedia/pdf/CG020NICEguideline.pdf

Chapter 4

Efficacy of ketogenic dietary therapy: what is the evidence?

Eric H. Kossoff

Johns Hopkins Hospital, Baltimore, Maryland, USA

Although used for nearly a century, there is still some level of belief amongst the child neurology community that the use of ketogenic diet (KD) is less proven than anticonvulsant medication. In comparison, there is certainly a relative dearth of randomized controlled trials, yet the evidence from often large retrospective studies is compelling. In this chapter, I discuss the clinical evidence that dietary therapies are effective.

How well does it work overall?

Since the diet has been available, many large studies have been published regarding its benefits (Table 4.1) (Henderson et al., 2006). These studies are nearly universally completed in children with intractable epilepsy, which makes the positive results even more impressive when evaluated. Studies go back nearly a century.

One of the earliest retrospective studies was by Peterman (1924) from the Mayo Clinic in Rochester, Minnesota. In this study including 17 children, 10 (60%) were seizure-free and four (23%) were significantly (>90%) improved. Few prospective or large studies followed over the next 70 years until 1998, when the largest prospective study up to that time was published (Freeman et al., 1998). In this study, 150 children aged 1–16 years with more than two seizures per week who had failed at least two anticonvulsants were followed for 1 year. At 6 months, 71% remained on the diet; 51% had a greater than 50% improvement and 32% had a greater than 90% reduction. No specific seizure type preferentially improved, but the diet was less effective in children older than 8 years.

In 2000, an article written for the United States Blue Cross Blue Shield insurance company reviewed all studies to date and concluded the diet led to a 'significant reduction in seizure frequency' and that 'it is unlikely that this degree of

Dietary Treatment of Epilepsy: Practical Implementation of Ketogenic Therapy,
First Edition. Edited by Elizabeth Neal.
© 2012 John Wiley & Sons, Ltd. Published 2012 by John Wiley & Sons, Ltd.

Table 4.1 A summary of selected published retrospective and prospective efficacy studies of the ketogenic diet including over 20 patients, 1990–present.

Reference	No. of patients	>90% improvement rate at 6 months	>50% improvement rate at 6 months
Kinsman et al. (1992)	58	29%	67%
Vining et al. (1998)*	51	29%	53%
Freeman et al. (1998)*	150	32%	51%
Hassan et al. (1999)	52		67%
Kankirawatana et al. (2001)*	35	75%	
Nordli et al. (2001)	32		55%
Coppola et al. (2002)*	56		27%
François et al. (2003)	29		41%
Mady et al. (2003)	45	29%	50%
Kim et al. (2004)	124	53% (3 months)	76% (3 months)
Klepper et al. (2004)	111	17%	31%
Vaisleib et al. (2004)	54		65%
Seo et al. (2007)	74	24%	79%
Neal et al. (2008)*	54	7%	38%
Nathan et al. (2009)*	105	62%	80%
Hong et al. (2010)*	104		64%
Dressler et al. (2010)	50	48%	50%

*Prospective studies.

benefit can result from a placebo response and/or spontaneous remission' (Lefevre and Aronson, 2000). In all studies combined, 16% were seizure-free, 32% improved by more than 90% and 56% improved by more than 50%. This is what we tell prospective parents. In general, approximately 50–60% of children will have 50% or more reduction in seizures, of whom 15% will become seizure-free (Figure 4.1). Most studies of anticonvulsants in children with recalcitrant seizures will demonstrate about half these response rates.

For years one of the main criticisms of the KD was the lack of randomized and controlled studies. A Cochrane Library meta-analysis in 2003 concluded 'there is no reliable evidence from randomized controlled trials to support the use of KDs for people with epilepsy' (Levy and Cooper, 2003). However, the reviewers judged the diet as a 'possible option' due to the observation that 'a small number of observational studies lend some support for a beneficial effect'.

The lack of randomized studies noted in 2003 is no longer accurate. A study randomizing patients to either a fasting period or gradual introduction of the diet by the Children's Hospital of Philadelphia revealed no long-term differences in efficacy but fewer side effects (Bergqvist et al., 2005). This study is often quoted as evidence that fasting is not required for long-term efficacy. However, retrospective evidence from Baltimore and Chicago suggests that in

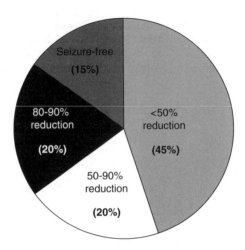

Figure 4.1   Efficacy of the ketogenic diet in multiple studies after 6 months of treatment.

the short term, a 24-hour fasting period will lead to a more rapid response to the KD, which can be reassuring to families and perhaps lead to a quicker anticonvulsant reduction (Kossoff et al., 2008a).

In 2008, a study examining the medium-chain triglyceride (MCT) and classical (long-chain triglyceride) diets was completed at Great Ormond Street Hospital in London (Neal et al., 2008) in which 145 children aged 2–16 years who had failed to respond to at least two appropriate anticonvulsants and had at least seven seizures weekly were randomized to receive a KD, either immediately or after a 3-month delay with anticonvulsants continued and no additional treatment changes (control group). Of the 73 children who were allocated to a KD and the 72 allocated to a control period, data from 103 were available for analysis (54 KD, 49 control). These investigators found that the seizure frequency after 3 months was significantly lower in the children on the diet (38% decrease in seizures) compared with the 49 control children (37% *increase* in seizures) ($P<0.0001$). Of the diet group, 28 had greater than 50% seizure reduction (38%), compared with four controls (6%) ($P<0.0001$), and one KD child achieved seizure freedom. No child in the control group had a greater than 90% reduction in seizures, compared with five on KD ($P=0.06$). The authors acknowledge that their responder rates, based on intention-to-treat analyses, are lower than many others (Table 4.1), and they suggest that this may be partly due to the very severe intractable nature of the seizures experienced by many of the children included in their trial, the possibility of selection bias occurring in some cohort studies, and the fact that their trial did not include children under the age of 2 years. No difference was seen in efficacy between the classical and MCT diets, the latter being also a randomized arm of this trial (Neal et al., 2009). Although this control group did not include a new treatment (e.g. an adjunctive anticonvulsant), the results clearly demonstrate that the KD is effective over continued observation and contradicts any argument that KD responses are solely due to the normal fluctuations in seizure frequency seen in epilepsy.

A randomized, double blind, placebo-controlled trial of 20 patients (60 g daily glucose versus saccharin solution given sequentially as a crossover during an initial fasting period) was completed at the Johns Hopkins Hospital that same year (Freeman et al., 2009). The blind was successful, with parents and investigators being unaware of which solution the child was given or their level of ketosis. Unfortunately, only a strong trend towards statistical significance was identified in favour of the saccharin (treatment) group over the glucose (placebo) group ($P = 0.07$). Overall there was a mean decrease of 34 seizures per day over the 12-day study period ($P = 0.003$). Likely reasons for the study not reaching statistical significance include insufficient glucose (and ketosis in the placebo group), the powerful effects of fasting in both groups, and too short a period allowed for return to a baseline level of seizure frequency during the crossover between the treatment arms. However, this study demonstrates that the KD can be studied in a blinded manner, previously deemed impossible.

Who should it be used for?

With regard to seizure type, the most common use of the diet is for children with symptomatic generalized epilepsies such as Lennox–Gastaut syndrome. This syndrome is one of the more common conditions to be investigated in both retrospective and prospective studies of the diet (Freeman et al., 2009). In this condition, children will often have multiple seizure types including atonic, tonic, myoclonic and atypical absence seizures. The electroencephalogram (EEG) will commonly reveal slow (2–2.5 Hz) spike–wave discharges with an abnormal background.

Other than Lennox–Gastaut syndrome, there was a belief in the child neurology community that all other children were equally likely to respond to the KD. This does not appear to be true based on the past decade of research. In fact, the initial table of the 2009 International Expert Consensus Guideline for the use of the KD is devoted to the 'indications' for which the KD is especially useful (Kossoff et al., 2009). The two most widely reported conditions include glucose transporter (GLUT) type 1 deficiency and pyruvate dehydrogenase (PDH) deficiency. Both conditions are metabolic ones in which the KD is the only therapy that treats the underlying condition. In these situations, seizures may be mild in fact.

What about other epilepsy conditions? Perhaps most promising is infantile spasms. In this condition, which affects infants aged 3–6 months at onset, a high-voltage, chaotic, multifocal spike and slow wave pattern is recognized on EEG in association with clusters of head drops and arm extensions. Infants often have developmental delay in association with this condition. Effective therapies include adrenocorticotrophin hormone (ACTH), prednisolone and vigabatrin, but all have significant side effects and at times cost issues. The KD appears to be very helpful for intractable infantile spasms (Hong et al., 2010). In this large study of 104 infants, about two-thirds of children (64%) with this condition had at least a 50% or more decrease in their spasms within 6 months of treatment, of which 38 (37%) became spasm-free for at least 6 months (Hong et al., 2010). As a result of this growing evidence for intractable infantile spasms, our centre has used the KD in children for new-onset infantile spasms (if the family brings the child in within 2 weeks). Results to date are that 10 of 21 (47%) of infants become spasm-free within 2 weeks of treatment.

Other generalized seizure types such as myoclonic, atonic and tonic seizures have been treated effectively with the diet, especially those affecting infants or very young children. Myoclonic astatic epilepsy (Doose syndrome) has been reported to be amenable to the KD as well (Kilaru and Bergqvist, 2007). Most epileptologists do not believe the diet is as effective for partial (focal) onset epilepsy. In a study of 150 children placed on the diet by Johns Hopkins Hospital, the diet was equally effective for all seizure types, including partial epilepsy (Freeman et al., 1998); however, others have found it less effective. When 18 children who had an early dramatic response (seizure-free within 2 weeks) to the KD were compared with the overall population, none had partial epilepsy (Than et al., 2005). Our experience suggests that the KD is very helpful in managing partial onset epilepsy, and occasionally delays the time until resective surgery is performed, but rarely represents a cure. Data in children who specifically are surgical candidates have indicated this assessment is true (Stainman et al., 2007).

Other conditions for which the KD has been beneficial include tuberous sclerosis complex (TSC) and Rett syndrome (Kossoff et al., 2005). After 6 months, 11 (92%) of the combined 12 children treated with the diet for intractable seizures associated with TSC at Johns Hopkins Hospital and Massachusetts General Hospital were over 50% improved, and eight (67%) were more than 90% improved (Kossoff et al., 2005). Five children had seizure-free periods of at least 5 months' duration. For this syndrome, typically associated with focal epilepsy (due to cortical tubers), the efficacy was surprisingly high.

Another population worth discussion is children with epilepsy who have gastrostomy tubes in place for nutrition. Patients on formula-only diets have guaranteed compliance along with excellent tolerability. In a study from Johns Hopkins of 61 children formula-fed (30 had gastrostomy tubes), 59% had greater than 90% seizure reduction at 12 months, which is nearly double that of the overall population treated with the diet (Kossoff et al., 2004a).

Evidence for 'alternative' ketogenic diets

The modified Atkins diet (MAD) and low glycemic index treatment (LGIT) have also demonstrated short-term (generally 6 months) efficacy for intractable epilepsy. The MAD has also been studied in 26 prospective and retrospective studies to date (Kossoff et al., 2006; Kang et al., 2007; Kossoff and Dorward, 2008). Of the 347 children and adults who have been reported, 144 (41%) had a greater than 50% seizure reduction; 86 (25%) had greater than 90% seizure reduction, which is very similar to the percentage often quoted for the KD. Similar to the KD, when successful, the MAD works within 2–4 weeks. Recent long-term data suggests this benefit is maintained beyond 6 months (Chen and Kossoff, 2012).

The MAD appears to be helpful for adults as well (discussed below). In addition, it has been used in Honduras for a child with intractable seizures without access to a dietitian or KD center (Kossoff et al., 2008b). Similarly, it has been tried for non-epilepsy conditions such as migraine (Kossoff et al., 2010a).

Should the MAD not be as effective as desired, it is also theoretically possible for the family and KD centre to switch the child to the formal KD. In a recently completed multicentre retrospective study, 27 children switched from the MAD to the KD were examined (Kossoff et al., 2010b); 10 (37%) had greater than 10% seizure reduction with the additional switch and no child who did not respond to the MAD then responded to the KD, suggesting that the KD is likely a 'higher dose' of dietary therapy, but not unique. Interestingly, of the five children who became seizure-free with the switch (who were not before), all five had myoclonic astatic epilepsy (Doose syndrome). As a result of this study, we now routinely recommend switching to the KD for all children with Doose syndrome not seizure-free after 6–9 months of the MAD.

Two formal retrospective studies of the LGIT have been published, and 10 (50%) of 20 children had greater than 90% seizure reduction in the first (Pfeifer and Thiele, 2005). In 2009, the authors updated their results with a total of 76 children, with results after 1 month demonstrating a 50% reduction in seizures in approximately 50% of children (Muzykewicz et al., 2009). Similar to the MAD, ketosis did not correlate with seizure control, although serum ketone levels were higher than baseline at all time points. At 1 and 12 months on the LGIT, lower serum glucose levels were significantly associated with likelihood of greater than 90% seizure reduction.

Ages older than childhood

Adolescents have also been successfully managed with the KD, despite a common misperception that the diet is intolerable for children in high school due to social factors and restrictiveness. A retrospective study from Johns Hopkins Hospital and the University of Texas at Houston reported on 45 patients aged 12–19 years (Mady et al., 2003). Despite the concerns of possible restrictiveness, seizure improvement and tolerability were remarkably similar to those in more typical school-age children. After 12 months, 20 (44%) of 45 remained on the diet, with 13 (65%) achieving greater than 50% seizure reduction (Mady et al., 2003). Today, most teenagers are started on the MAD due to ease of use in that population, especially if the adolescent is cognitively normal and not gastrostomy-tube fed.

Although an apparently new concept, use of the KD for adults was described in the literature as early as 1930, where 100 adults were treated (Barborka, 1930). In this study from the Mayo Clinic, 56 % had a greater than 50 % response and 12 % were seizure-free, an outcome remarkably similar to that reported for children. Although not systematically monitored, cholesterol increased in several patients; amenorrhoea occurred in 12 (21 %) of the 56 women treated, an occurrence also seen in the study of adolescents (Mady et al., 2003).

With the advent of new anticonvulsants, it took many years for the KD to be studied again in adults. In 1999, the group in Philadelphia studied 19 adults, of whom 54 % had a greater than 50 % response, and the 12 patients with symptomatic generalized epilepsy had the best outcome, with 73 % having a greater than 50 % response compared with only 27 % of the 11 adults with partial epilepsy (Sirven et al., 1999). Diet duration was relatively short for these adults (7 months average). Weight loss was notable, with a mean decrease of 6.7 kg. The traditional KD has also been recently studied in adults with similar results from Israel and the USA (see Chapter 23).

Early in the use of the MAD, it was believed to be a potentially very helpful treatment over the KD for adults. A prospective trial of MAD (15 g of carbohydrates per day, with encouragement of fat intake) for adults was then completed in 2008 (Kossoff et al., 2008c). In 30 patients prospectively started on the MAD with 15 g of carbohydrates per day, 47 % had seizure reduction after 1 and 3 months and 33 % after 6 months. Interestingly, a decrease in weight as measured by the body mass index seemed to correlate with seizure control, but only at the 3-month visit ($P=0.03$). Cholesterol, urine calcium and blood urea nitrogen did increase.

Efficacy beyond seizure control

Other than seizure reduction, many parents request other benefits. Perhaps the most common is medication reduction, for side effects as well as costs. Data would suggest that anticonvulsants can be successfully reduced even during the diet initiation period, although we typically suggest waiting a month (Kossoff et al., 2004b). In addition, parents request and may see cognitive improvement in their children, although this is difficult to differentiate from seizure and medication reduction (Farasat et al., 2006). In fact, this latter request is the most associated with total time on the KD, perhaps indicating that for parents it is the most important outcome.

Summary

The evidence for benefits of the KD is extensive. In both retrospective as well as recent randomized and controlled studies, approximately half of children with intractable epilepsy have significant seizure reduction. In addition, alternative diets such as the MAD and LGIT appear efficacious. Beyond childhood, these diets can lead to seizure reduction in adolescents and adults as well. Proven today, the use of dietary therapy is popular, powerful and here to stay.

References

Barborka, C.J. (1930) Epilepsy in adults: results of treatment by ketogenic diet in one hundred cases. *Arch Neurol* **6**, 904–914.

Bergqvist, A.G., Schall, J.I., Gallagher, P.R., Cnaan, A. and Stallings, V.A. (2005) Fasting versus gradual initiation of the ketogenic diet: a prospective, randomized clinical trial of efficacy. *Epilepsia* **46**, 1810–1819.

Coppola, G., Veggiotti, P., Cusmai, R. et al. (2002) The ketogenic diet in children, adolescents and young adults with refractory epilepsy: an Italian multi-centre experience. *Epilepsy Res* **48**, 221–227.

Chen, W. and Kossoff, E.H. (2012) Long-term follow-up of children treated with the Modified Atkins Diet. *J Child Neurol* (in press).

Dressler, A., Stöcklin, B., Reithofer, E. et al. (2010) Long-term outcome and tolerability of the ketogenic diet in drug-resistant childhood epilepsy: the Austrian experience. *Seizure* **19**, 404–408.

Farasat, S., Kossoff, E.H., Pillas, D.J., Rubenstein, J.E., Vining, E.P. and Freeman, J.M. (2006) The importance of cognition in parental expectations prior to starting the ketogenic diet. *Epilepsy Behav* **8**, 406–410.

François, L.L., Manel, V., Rousselle, C. and David, M. (2003) Ketogenic regime as anti-epileptic treatment: its use in 29 epileptic children [French]. *Arch Pediatr* **10**, 300–306.

Freeman, J.M., Vining, E.P.G., Pillas, D.J., Pyzik, P.L., Casey, J.C. and Kelly, M.T. (1998) The efficacy of the ketogenic diet 1998: a prospective evaluation of intervention in 150 children. *Pediatrics* **102**, 1358–1363.

Freeman, J.M., Vining, E.P.G., Kossoff, E.H., Pyzik, P.L., Ye, X. and Goodman, S.N. (2009) A blinded, crossover study of the ketogenic diet. *Epilepsia* **50**, 322–325.

Hassan, A.M., Keene, D.L., Whiting, S.E., Jacob, P.J., Champagne, J.R. and Humphreys, P. (1999) Ketogenic diet in the treatment of refractory epilepsy in childhood. *Pediatr Neurol* **21**, 548–552.

Henderson, C.B., Filloux, F.M., Alder, S.C., Lyon, J.L. and Caplin, D.A. (2006) Efficacy of the ketogenic diet as a treatment option for epilepsy: meta-analysis. *J Child Neurol* **21**, 193–198.

Hong, A.M., Hamdy, R.F., Turner, Z. and Kossoff, E.H. (2010) Infantile spasms treated with the ketogenic diet: prospective single-center experience in 104 consecutive infants. *Epilepsia* **51**, 1403–1407.

Kang, H.C., Lee, H.S., You, S.J., Kang, Du C, Ko T.S. and Kim, H.D. (2007) Use of a modified Atkins diet in intractable childhood epilepsy. *Epilepsia* **48**, 182–186.

Kankirawatana, P., Jirapinyo, P., Kankirawatana, S., Wongarn, R. and Thamanasari, N. (2001) Ketogenic diet: an alternative treatment for refractory epilepsy in children. *J Med Assoc Thailand* **84**, 1027–1032.

Kilaru, S. and Bergqvist, A.G. (2007) Current treatment of myoclonic astatic epilepsy: clinical experience at the Children's Hospital of Philadelphia. *Epilepsia* **48**, 1703–1707.

Kim, D.W., Kang, H.C., Park, J.C. and Kim, H.D. (2004) Benefits of the nonfasting ketogenic diet compared with the initial fasting ketogenic diet. *Pediatrics* **114**, 1627–1630.

Kinsman, S.L., Vining, E.P.G., Quaskey, S.A., Mellitis, D. and Freeman, J.M. (1992) Efficacy of the ketogenic diet for intractable seizure disorders: review of 58 cases. *Epilepsia* **33**, 1132–1136.

Klepper, J., Leiendecker, B., Riemann, E. and Baumeister, F.A. (2004) The ketogenic diet in German-speaking countries: update 2003 [German]. *Klin Padiatr* **216**, 277–285.

Kossoff, E.H. and Dorward, J.L. (2008) The Modified Atkins Diet. *Epilepsia* **49**, 37–41.

Kossoff, E.H., McGrogan, J.R. and Freeman, J.M. (2004a) Benefits of an all-liquid ketogenic diet. *Epilepsia* **45**, 1163.

Kossoff, E.H., Pyzik, P.L., McGrogan, J.R. and Rubenstein, J.E. (2004b) Impact of early versus late anticonvulsant reduction after ketogenic diet initiation. *Epilepsy Behav* **5**, 499–502.

Kossoff, E.H., Thiele, E.A., Pfeifer, H.H., McGrogan, J.R. and Freeman, J.M. (2005) Tuberous sclerosis complex and the ketogenic diet. *Epilepsia* **46**, 1684–1686.

Kossoff, E.H., McGrogan, J.R., Bluml, R.M., Pillas, D.J., Rubenstein, J.E. and Vining, E.P. (2006) A modified Atkins diet is effective for the treatment of intractable pediatric epilepsy. *Epilepsia* **47**, 421–424.

Kossoff, E.H., Laux, L.C., Blackford, R. et al. (2008a) When do seizures improve with the ketogenic diet? *Epilepsia* **49**, 329–333.

Kossoff, E.H., Dorward, J.L., Molinero, M.R. and Holden, K.R. (2008b) The Modified Atkins Diet: a potential treatment for developing countries. *Epilepsia* **49**, 1646–1647.

Kossoff, E.H., Rowley, H., Sinha, S.R. and Vining, E.P.G. (2008c) A prospective study of the modified Atkins diet for intractable epilepsy in adults. *Epilepsia* **49**, 316–319.

Kossoff, E.H., Zupec-Kania, B.A., Amark, P.E. et al. (2009) Optimal clinical management of children receiving the ketogenic diet: recommendations of the international ketogenic diet study group. *Epilepsia* **50**, 304–317.

Kossoff, E.H., Huffman, J., Turner, Z. and Gladstein, J. (2010a) Use of the modified Atkins diet for adolescents with chronic daily headache. *Cephalalgia* **30**, 1014–1016.

Kossoff, E.H., Dorward, J.L., Miranda, M.J., Wiemer-Kruel, A., Kang, H.C. and Kim, H.D. (2010b) Will seizure control improve by switching from the Modified Atkins Diet to the traditional ketogenic diet? *Epilepsia* **51**, 2496–2499.

Lefevre, F. and Aronson, N. (2000) Ketogenic diet for the treatment of refractory epilepsy in children: a systematic review of efficacy. *Pediatrics* **105**, e46.

Levy, R. and Cooper, P. (2003) Ketogenic diet for epilepsy. *Cochrane Database Syst Rev* (**3**), CD001903.

Mady, M.A., Kossoff, E.H., McGregor, A.L., Wheless, J.W., Pyzik, P.L. and Freeman, J.M. (2003) The ketogenic diet: adolescents can do it, too. *Epilepsia* **44**, 847–851.

Muzykewicz, D.A., Lyczkowski, D.A., Memon, N., Conant, K.D., Pfeifer, H.H. and Thiele, E.A. (2009) Efficacy, safety, and tolerability of the low glycemic index treatment in pediatric epilepsy. *Epilepsia* **50**, 1118–1126.

Nathan, J.K., Purandare, A.S., Parekh, Z.B. and Manohar, H.V. (2009) Ketogenic diet in Indian children with uncontrolled epilepsy. *Indian Pediatr* **46**, 669–673.

Neal, E.G., Chaffe, H., Schwartz, R.H. et al. (2008) The ketogenic diet for the treatment of childhood epilepsy: a randomised controlled trial. *Lancet Neurol* **7**, 500–506.

Neal, E.G., Chaffe, H.M., Schwartz, R. et al. (2009) A randomised trial of classical and medium-chain triglyceride ketogenic diets in the treatment of childhood epilepsy. *Epilepsia* **50**, 1109–1117.

Nordli, D.R. Jr, Kuroda, M.M., Carroll, J. et al. (2001) Experience with the ketogenic diet in infants. *Pediatrics* **108**, 129–133.

Peterman, M.G. (1924) The ketogenic diet in the treatment of epilepsy: a preliminary report. *Am J Dis Child* **28**, 28–33.

Pfeifer, H.H. and Thiele, E.A. (2005) Low glycemic-index treatment: a liberalized ketogenic diet for treatment of intractable epilepsy. *Neurology* **65**, 1810–1812.

Seo, J.H., Lee, Y.M., Lee, J.S., Kang, H.C. and Kim, H.D. (2007) Efficacy and tolerability of the ketogenic diet according to lipid:nonlipid ratios: comparison of 3:1 with 4:1 diet. *Epilepsia* **48**, 801–805.

Sirven, J., Whedon, B., Caplan, D. et al. (1999) The ketogenic diet for intractable epilepsy in adults: preliminary results. *Epilepsia* **40**, 1721–1726.

Stainman, R.S., Turner, Z., Rubenstein, J.E. and Kossoff, E.H. (2007) Decreased relative efficacy of the ketogenic diet for children with surgically approachable epilepsy. *Seizure* **16**, 615–619.

Than, K.D., Kossoff, E.H., Rubenstein, J.E., Pyzik, P.L., McGrogan, J.R. and Vining, E.P.G. (2005) Can you predict an immediate, complete, and sustained response to the ketogenic diet? *Epilepsia* **46**, 580–582.

Vaisleib, I.I., Buchalter, J.R. and Zupanc, M.L. (2004). Ketogenic diet: outpatient initiation, without fluid or caloric restrictions. *Pediatr Neurol* **31**, 198–202.

Vining, E.P.G., Freeman, J.M., Ballaban-Gil, K. et al. (1998) A multi-center study of the efficacy of the ketogenic diet. *Arch Neurol* **55**, 1433–1437.

Chapter 5

The biochemical basis of dietary therapies for neurological disorders

Adam L. Hartman[1] and Jong M. Rho[2]

[1]*Johns Hopkins Hospital, Baltimore, Maryland, USA*
[2]*University of Calgary Faculty of Medicine and Alberta Children's Hospital, Calgary, Alberta, Canada*

The most prominent example of an effective metabolic treatment for epilepsy is the high-fat, low-carbohydrate ketogenic diet (KD), which has been used for nearly a century to treat infants and children with medically intractable epilepsy. The KD is so named because the high-fat content produces a fundamental biochemical shift away from glucose utilization (i.e. glycolysis) to fatty acid oxidation and hence the production of ketone bodies, notably β-hydroxybutyrate (BHB), acetoacetate and acetone. How such changes influence neuronal cellular activity and integrity remains unclear, but research in this area has been rapidly accelerating. Importantly, insights gleaned about KD effects at molecular, cellular and genetic levels are prerequisites for implementing rational strategies to improve the efficacy of this unique treatment and to enhance tolerability. This chapter highlights the major biochemical features of currently employed dietary treatments for epilepsy and focuses on the principal metabolic changes induced by the KD and its variants. The reader is referred to other recent sources for more detailed information (Bough and Rho, 2007; Hartman et al., 2007; Masino and Rho, 2012).

Components of different diets

Different types of KDs are commonly used in the clinic. The first consists largely of long-chain saturated fatty acids – the 'classical' KD (Hartman and Vining, 2007). An alternative consists of large amounts of medium-chain triglycerides (MCT), either from dietary sources such as coconut oil or commercially available oil preparations – the 'MCT diet' (Huttenlocher et al., 1971). Metabolism of

---

Dietary Treatment of Epilepsy: Practical Implementation of Ketogenic Therapy,
First Edition. Edited by Elizabeth Neal.
© 2012 John Wiley & Sons, Ltd. Published 2012 by John Wiley & Sons, Ltd.

both diets is reviewed but some details will be omitted for the sake of clarity. Two recent reviews provide excellent source material on the topic of fat metabolism (Salway, 2004; Ratnayake and Galli, 2009).

Fat absorption and metabolism

Fat from dietary sources typically comprises a blend of fatty acids with varying chain lengths (long, medium and short chain). Fatty acids are emulsified and then digested by lipases secreted through the upper gastrointestinal tract. Short- and medium-chain fatty acids are absorbed through the gastric and intestinal lining into the bloodstream, where they bind to albumin. Long-chain fatty acids become one component of micelles and diffuse into enterocytes, where they are incorporated into the endoplasmic reticulum, activated to coenzyme A (CoA) derivatives by the cofactor acyl-CoA, and then converted into triglycerides. Triglycerides are then transported out of enterocytes into the lymphatic system, and subsequently into venous blood as one component of a chylomicron. Within the chylomicron, triglycerides are hydrolysed to free fatty acids and glycerol, which can be used by cells or stored in adipose tissue. Some free fatty acids bind to albumin.

Free fatty acids bound to albumin can be taken into hepatocytes via the portal circulation. Fatty acids form acyl-CoA derivatives (via long-chain acyl-CoA synthetase). Very long chain fatty acids undergo initial metabolism via β-oxidation in peroxisomes. Metabolism of short-, medium- and long-chain fatty acids proceeds primarily through mitochondrial β-oxidation. Cytosolic fatty acids are transported across the outer mitochondrial membrane-bound carnitine-palmitoyl transferase I and inner mitochondrial membrane-bound carnitine-palmitoyl transferase II and carnitine/acylcarnitine translocase. Fatty acids then undergo metabolism initially via acyl-CoA dehydrogenases, with the net production of acetyl-CoA and other fatty acids, which eventually become backbones for prostaglandins, leukotrienes, resolvins, protectins or other fatty acid derivatives, including cell membrane and vesicular components (Phillis et al., 2006; Levy, 2010). Some of these derivatives include polyunsaturated fatty acids (PUFAs), which also exert regulatory effects (discussed below).

Ketone bodies can be generated from fatty acids. Initially, two acetyl-CoA molecules form acetoacetyl-CoA via the acetoacetyl-CoA thiolase reaction, with a third acetyl-CoA attached via 3-hydroxy-3-methylglutaryl (HMG)-CoA synthase, yielding HMG-CoA. Cleavage of HMG-CoA yields acetoacetate and acetyl-CoA, some of which is reduced to BHB (or D-3-hydroxybutyrate). Some of the acetoacetate is also spontaneously decarboxylated to form acetone, which may eventually be exhaled via the lungs or undergo further metabolism into acetyl-CoA and oxaloacetate. Ketone bodies can also be formed from amino acids, including isoleucine (acetyl-CoA), leucine (HMG-CoA), lysine and tryptophan (acetoacetyl-CoA), and phenylalanine and tyrosine (acetoacetate). Although typically considered a process that only

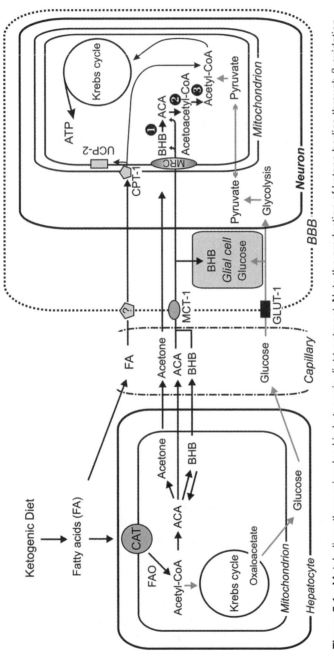

Figure 5.1 Metabolic pathways involved in ketogenic diet treatment. Note the production of ketone bodies through β-oxidation in the liver, release and transport through the systemic circulation, transport past the blood–brain barrier via a monocarboxylic acid transporter (MCT)-1, entry into brain mitochondria and conversion into substrates for tricarboxylic acid (Krebs) cycle function. ACA, acetoacetate; ATP, adenosine triphosphate; BBB, blood–brain barrier; BHB, β-hydroxybutyrate; CAT, carnitine-acylcarnitine translocase; CPT-1, carnitine palmitoyltransferase; FAO, fatty acid oxidation; GLUT-1, glucose transporter 1; MRC, mitochondrial respiratory complex; UCP, uncoupling protein; 1, 3-hydroxybutyrate dehydrogenase; 2, succinyl-CoA–3-oxoacid-CoA transferase; 3, mitochondrial acetoacetyl-CoA thiolase. From Kim Do and Rho (2008). Used with permission from Worters Kluwer Health.

occurs in the liver, there is evidence that astrocytes can generate ketone bodies under certain conditions (Blazquez et al., 1999).

Under certain physiological states (e.g. fasting or extreme stress) fuels other than glucose can be used, including ketone bodies. Ketone bodies cannot be used by hepatocytes (because they lack 3-ketoacyl-CoA) but are utilized by other cells. In the brain, ketone bodies are transported across vascular endothelial cells via the monocarboxylate transporter (MCT-1). After entry into neurones, glia and other cells, BHB is metabolized in mitochondria to acetoacetate by the inner membrane-bound enzyme BHB dehydrogenase. Succinyl-CoA serves as a donor to form acetoacetyl-CoA via 3-ketoacyl-CoA transferase. Cleavage of acetoacetyl-CoA yields two acetyl-CoAs via acetoacetyl-CoA thiolase. Acetyl-CoA can then be used in the Krebs cycle to form adenosine triphosphate (ATP). The Krebs cycle also produces α-ketoglutarate, which is converted to the excitatory amino acid glutamate via glutamate dehydrogenase. In turn, glutamate can be converted via glutamate decarboxylase into γ-aminobutyric acid (GABA), the primary inhibitory neurotransmitter in the mammalian brain. The principal steps beginning with fatty acid ingestion, oxidation and breakdown in the liver, systemic transport, entry into brain and subsequent conversion to Krebs cycle substrates are summarized in Figure 5.1.

Mechanisms of action of ketogenic diet

The mechanisms underlying the clinical effects of the KD are not fully understood, but likely involve multiple parallel (and possibly) synergistic mechanisms resulting in an anticonvulsant, and possibly neuroprotective, effect (Figure 5.2).

Glycolysis, ketone bodies and Krebs cycle function

BHB is the major ketone body formed by the liver during ketogenesis and has been traditionally followed in the clinical setting to assess the degree of fatty acid oxidation. Based on current evidence, the clinical efficacy of the KD does not appear to correlate with blood levels of ketone bodies. Interestingly, however, both acetoacetate and acetone (but not BHB) have been shown to be directly anticonvulsant when administered intraperitoneally in laboratory animals (Rho et al., 2002). Such data might predict that ketone bodies would reduce neuronal hyperexcitability and/or hypersynchrony, but thus far *in vitro* experiments have failed to demonstrate this (Thio et al., 2000). Taken together, the available evidence would suggest that the effects of the KD may not be a direct anticonvulsant effect of ketone bodies, but rather a reflection of a larger systemic adaptation – marked by ketosis – as patients shift their metabolism to reduced glycolytic flux and increased fatty acid oxidation.

Another characteristic feature of the KD is lowered glucose levels during clinical treatment. Glucose restriction alone may play an important role in an

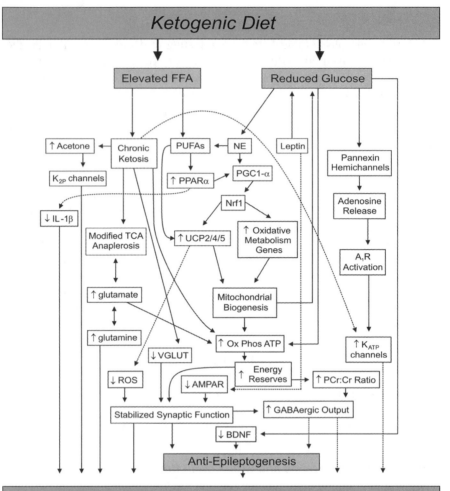

Figure 5.2 Hypothetical pathways leading to the anticonvulsant effects of the ketogenic diet. Elevated free fatty acids (FFA) lead to chronic ketosis and increased concentrations of polyunsaturated fatty acids (PUFAs) in the brain. Chronic ketosis is predicted to lead to increased levels of acetone; this might activate K_{2P} channels to hyperpolarize neurones and limit neuronal excitability. Chronic ketosis is also anticipated to modify the tricarboxylic acid (TCA) cycle, as would the presence of anaplerotic substrates such as triheptanoin. This would increase glutamate and, subsequently, GABA synthesis in the brain. Among several direct inhibitory actions, PUFAs boost the activity of brain-specific uncoupling proteins (UCPs). This is expected to limit generation of reactive oxygen species (ROS), neuronal dysfunction and resultant neurodegeneration. Acting via the nuclear transcription factor peroxisome proliferator-activated receptor (PPAR)-α and its co-activator peroxisome proliferator-activated receptor γ coactivator-1 (PGC-1α), PUFAs would induce the expression of UCPs and coordinately upregulate several dozen genes related to oxidative energy metabolism. PPARα expression is inversely correlated with interleukin (IL)-1β cytokine expression; given the role of IL-1β in hyperexcitability and

anticonvulsant action of the KD, as evidenced by several studies (Maalouf et al., 2009). Calorie restriction in rodents reduced seizure susceptibility and lowered levels of blood glucose, which correlated with inhibition of epileptogenesis. These data indicate that less readily available glucose may limit the brain's ability to generate and promote seizure activity. Other investigators have postulated a more direct effect of glucose restriction through a reduction/diversion of glycolytic flux (Garriga-Canut et al., 2006; Lian et al., 2007). Further, the concept that ketones may be directly anticonvulsant has been resurrected, either through activation of potassium channels (Ma et al., 2007; Kawamura et al., 2010) which largely function to dampen excitation, or by preventing excitatory glutamate release through an interaction with vesicular glutamate transporters or VGLUTs (Juge et al., 2010), despite earlier evidence to the contrary (Thio et al., 2000). Further downstream the metabolic cascade, the concept that refilling of Krebs cycle substrates through a process known as 'anaplerosis' (evoked by ingestion of the anaplerotic compound triheptanoin) may be effective has been validated in animal seizure models (Willis et al., 2010).

Polyunsaturated fatty acids

While ketone bodies have historically received much attention given the KD name, fatty acids are also likely critically involved in anticonvulsant activity. It is

Figure 5.2 (cont'd)   seizure generation, diminished expression of IL-1β cytokines during KD treatment could lead to improved seizure control. Ultimately, PUFAs would stimulate mitochondrial biogenesis. Mitochondrial biogenesis is predicted to increase ATP production capacity and enhance energy reserves, leading to stabilized synaptic function and improved seizure control. In particular, an elevated phosphocreatine/creatine (PCr:Cr) energy-reserve ratio is predicted to enhance GABAergic output, perhaps in conjunction with the ketosis-induced elevated GABA production, leading to diminished hyperexcitability. Reduced glucose coupled with elevated free fatty acids are proposed to reduce glycolytic flux during KD, which would further be feedback inhibited by high concentrations of citrate and ATP produced during KD treatment. This would activate metabolic K_{ATP} channels. Ketones may also directly activate K_{ATP} channels. Reduced glucose alone under conditions of adequate or enhanced energy levels activate pannexin hemichannels on CA3 pyramidal neurones, releasing ATP into the extracellular space; ATP is converted via ectonucleotidases to adenosine which subsequently activates adenosine receptors (A_1R). A_1R activation is also coupled to K_{ATP} channels. Ultimately, opening of K_{ATP} channels would hyperpolarize neurones and diminish neuronal excitability to contribute to the anticonvulsant (and perhaps neuroprotective) actions of the KD. Increased leptin, seen with KD treatment, can reduce glucose levels and inhibit AMPA (α-amino-3-hydroxy-5-methyl-4-isoxazolepropionic acid) receptor-mediated synaptic excitation. Reduced glucose is also expected to downregulate brain-derived neurotrophic factor (BDNF) and TrkB signalling in brain. As activation of TrkB pathways by BDNF has been shown to promote hyperexcitability and kindling, these potential KD-induced effects would be expected to limit the symptom (seizures) as well as epileptogenesis. Boxed variables depict findings described from KD studies; up (↑) or down (↓) arrows indicate the direction of the relationship between variables as a result of KD treatment. Dashed lines are used to clarify linkages and are not meant to suggest either magnitude or relative importance compared with solid lines. Adapted from Masino and Rho (2012). Used with permission from Oxford University Press.

well known that PUFAs can directly inhibit voltage-gated Na^+ and Ca^{2+} channels, but the relevance of these *in vitro* effects remains unclear (Leaf, 2001). Notwithstanding the challenge in linking *in vitro* findings to *in vivo* effects, PUFAs may mediate anticonvulsant effects through peroxisome proliferator-activated receptors (PPARs), which are highly linked to many of the biochemical changes associated with KD treatment (see below; Wu et al., 1999; Cullingford, 2008). PUFAs may also exert a neuroprotective action through upregulation of mitochondrial uncoupling protein activity and expression (Sullivan et al., 2004), which can decrease the production of damaging reactive oxygen species (ROS). Elevations in ROS have been implicated in the epileptic brain, as well as a variety of neurodegenerative conditions, including Alzheimer and Parkinson diseases, and amyotrophic lateral sclerosis (Patten et al., 2010).

Mitochondria and bioenergetics

The KD has also been reported to increase mitochondrial biogenesis and thus enhance overall availability of bioenergetic substrates (such as ATP), which may help stabilize cellular membrane function in the face of the metabolic stress that accompanies seizure activity (Bough et al., 2006). Specifically, elevations in ATP may help the functioning of the Na^+/K^+-ATPase, which would stabilize the neuronal cell membrane, hence limiting neuronal hyperexcitability and increasing the seizure threshold (Bough and Rho, 2007).

Neurotransmitter systems

Altered neurotransmitter function may play another critical role in the anticonvulsant effects of the KD. Norepinephrine levels are increased in brains of rats fed a KD, while mice lacking the ability to produce norepinephrine (i.e. dopamine-β-hydroxylase knockout mice) lose the protective benefits of the KD against seizures acutely provoked by fluorothyl, a volatile convulsant (Szot et al., 2001). More relevant to seizure control, levels of GABA may be increased by KD treatment (Yudkoff et al., 2008). Consistent with this notion, animal models of epilepsy induced by GABA antagonists have the strongest response to the KD (Uhlemann and Neims, 1972; Bough and Eagles, 1999), while clinical studies have demonstrated increased levels of GABA in the cerebrospinal fluid of patients, as have studies using magnetic resonance spectroscopy (Wang et al., 2003; Dahlin et al., 2005).

Regulators of metabolism

Glucose is the preferred fuel for cells under most circumstances. Glucose uptake into hepatocytes, muscle cells and fat cells is mediated by insulin, which is an anabolic hormone. Insulin also leads to increased fatty acid synthesis and esterification, as well as a decrease in lipolysis. In addition to lowering insulin levels in rodents (data in humans are mixed: Ross et al., 1985; Schwartz et al., 1989), the KD raises the level of leptin, an appetite-suppressing hormone produced predominantly in white adipose tissue (Thio et al., 2006). Leptin receptors are found in the hypothalamus (the most likely site of its central appetite-suppressing action) but also exist in hippocampus, neocortex and cerebellum (Harvey, 2007). Importantly, leptin has been shown to possess potent anticonvulsant effects (Xu et al., 2008).

One of the main regulators of fatty acid metabolism is PPARα, a nuclear hormone receptor and transcription factor (Cullingford, 2008). PPARα is activated by fatty acids (including PUFAs) and, in turn, increases fatty acid oxidation and generation of ketone bodies. Glucose also regulates PPARα activity. A related protein, PPARγ, is critical to function in brown fat and its cofactor, PGC-1α, is a master regulator of genes responsible for mitochondrial biogenesis and respiration (Wu et al., 1999).

Another mediator or 'sensor' of cellular metabolism is the mammalian target of rapamycin (mTOR) pathway. One component of this pathway (i.e. the RAPTOR complex) receives input signals from the insulin receptor and AMP-dependent protein kinase (AMPK), which in turn is responsive to conditions including hypoglycaemia, fasting, low ATP concentrations and high AMP levels (Laplante and Sabatini, 2009). In turn, this pathway influences fat metabolism and synthesis, protein synthesis, and translation (among other processes). Recently, the KD was shown to inhibit mTOR signalling in normal rodent brain (McDaniel et al., 2011).

Conclusion

While clinical data clearly demonstrate that the KD works, the underlying anticonvulsant (and possibly neuroprotective) mechanisms remain elusive. Nevertheless, metabolic treatments for epilepsy appear to have emerged from the shadow of empiricism and into the forefront of 'novel' therapeutic options. This is in large measure a consequence of concerted efforts on the part of both clinicians and researchers to investigate the neurobiological basis for KD action. A detailed understanding of relevant KD mechanisms could ultimately provide the scientific basis for developing a 'diet in a pill' (Rho and Sankar, 2008). The ultimate success of such initiatives depends heavily upon a firm grounding in biochemistry and pathophysiological disease processes.

Acknowledgements

Supported by the National Institutes of Health Clinician-Scientist Award 1K08NS070931 (A.L.H.) and 1RO1NS070261 (J.M.R.).

References

Blazquez, C., Woods, A., De Ceballos, M.L., Carling, D. and Guzman, M. (1999) The AMP-activated protein kinase is involved in the regulation of ketone body production by astrocytes. *J Neurochem* **73**, 1674–1682.

Bough, K.J. and Eagles, D.A. (1999) A ketogenic diet increases the resistance to pentylenetetrazole-induced seizures in the rat. *Epilepsia* **40**, 138–143.

Bough, K.J. and Rho, J.M. (2007) Anticonvulsant mechanisms of the ketogenic diet. *Epilepsia* **48**, 43–58.

Bough, K.J., Wetherington, J., Hassel, B. et al. (2006) Mitochondrial biogenesis in the anticonvulsant mechanism of the ketogenic diet. *Ann Neurol* **60**, 223–235.

Cullingford, T. (2008) Peroxisome proliferator-activated receptor alpha and the ketogenic diet. *Epilepsia* **49** (Suppl. 8), 70–72.

Dahlin, M., Elfving, A., Ungerstedt, U. and Amark, P. (2005) The ketogenic diet influences the levels of excitatory and inhibitory amino acids in the CSF in children with refractory epilepsy. *Epilepsy Res* **64**, 115–125.

Garriga-Canut, M., Schoenike, B., Qazi, R. et al. (2006) 2-Deoxy-D-glucose reduces epilepsy progression by NRSF-CtBP-dependent metabolic regulation of chromatin structure. *Nat Neurosci* **9**, 1382–1387.

Hartman, A.L. and Vining, E.P. (2007) Clinical aspects of the ketogenic diet. *Epilepsia* **48**, 31–42.

Hartman, A.L., Gasior, M., Vining, E.P. and Rogawski, M.A. (2007) The neuropharmacology of the ketogenic diet. *Pediatr Neurol* **36**, 281–292.

Harvey, J. (2007) Leptin: a diverse regulator of neuronal function. *J Neurochem* **100**, 307–313.

Huttenlocher, P.R., Wilbourn, A.J. and Signore, J.M. (1971) Medium-chain triglycerides as a therapy for intractable childhood epilepsy. *Neurology* **21**, 1097–1103.

Juge, N., Gray, J.A., Omote, H. et al. (2010) Metabolic control of vesicular glutamate transport and release. *Neuron* **68**, 99–112.

Kawamura, M. Jr, Ruskin, D.N. and Masino, S.A. (2010) Metabolic autocrine regulation of neurons involves cooperation among pannexin hemichannels, adenosine receptors, and KATP channels. *J Neurosci* **30**, 3886–3895.

Kim Do, Y. and Rho, J.M. (2008) The ketogenic diet and epilepsy. *Curr Opin Clin Nutr Metab Care* **11**, 113–120.

Laplante, M. and Sabatini, D.M. (2009) mTOR signaling at a glance. *J Cell Sci* **122**, 3589–3594.

Leaf, A. (2001) The electrophysiologic basis for the antiarrhythmic and anticonvulsant effects of n-3 polyunsaturated fatty acids: heart and brain. *Lipids* **36** (Suppl.), S107–S110.

Levy, B.D. (2010) Resolvins and protectins: natural pharmacophores for resolution biology. *Prostaglandins Leukot Essent Fatty Acids* **82**, 327–332.

Lian, X.Y., Khan, F.A. and Stringer, J.L. (2007) Fructose-1,6-bisphosphate has anticonvulsant activity in models of acute seizures in adult rats. *J Neurosci* **27**, 12007–12011.

Ma, W., Berg, J. and Yellen, G. (2007) Ketogenic diet metabolites reduce firing in central neurons by opening K(ATP) channels. *J Neurosci* **27**, 3618–3625.

Maalouf, M., Rho, J.M. and Mattson, M.P. (2009) The neuroprotective properties of calorie restriction, the ketogenic diet, and ketone bodies. *Brain Res Rev* **59**, 293–315.

McDaniel, S.S., Rensing, N.R., Thio, L.L., Yamada, K.A. and Wong, M. (2011) The ketogenic diet inhibits the mammalian target of rapamycin (mTOR) pathway. *Epilepsia* **52**, e7–11.

Masino, S.A. and Rho, J.M. (2012) Mechanisms of ketogenic diet action. In: Noebels, J.L., Avoli, M., Rogawski, M.A., Olsen, R.W. and Delgado-Escueta, A.V. (eds) *Jasper's Basic Mechanisms of the Epilepsies*, 4th edn. Oxford University Press.

Patten, D.A., Germain, M., Kelly, M.A. and Slack, R.S. (2010) Reactive oxygen species: stuck in the middle of neurodegeneration. *J Alzheimers Dis* **20** (Suppl. 2), S357–S367.

Phillis, J.W., Horrocks, L.A. and Farooqui, A.A. (2006) Cyclooxygenases, lipoxygenases, and epoxygenases in CNS: their role and involvement in neurological disorders. *Brain Res Rev* **52**, 201–243.

Ratnayake, W.M. and Galli, C. (2009) Fat and fatty acid terminology, methods of analysis and fat digestion and metabolism: a background review paper. *Ann Nutr Metab* **55**, 8–43.

Rho, J.M. and Sankar, R. (2008) The ketogenic diet in a pill: is this possible? *Epilepsia* **49** (Suppl. 8), 127–133.

Rho, J.M., Anderson, G.D., Donevan, S.D. and White, H.S. (2002) Acetoacetate, acetone, and dibenzylamine (a contaminant in l-(+)-beta-hydroxybutyrate) exhibit direct anticonvulsant actions in vivo. *Epilepsia* **43**, 358–361.

Ross, D.L., Swaiman, K.F., Torres, F. and Hansen, J. (1985) Early biochemical and EEG correlates of the ketogenic diet in children with atypical absence epilepsy. *Pediatr Neurol* **1**, 104–108.

Salway, J. (2004) *Metabolism at a Glance*. Oxford: Wiley-Blackwell.

Schwartz, R.M., Boyes, S. and Aynsley-Green, A. (1989) Metabolic effects of three ketogenic diets in the treatment of severe epilepsy. *Dev Med Child Neurol* **31**, 152–160.

Sullivan, P.G., Rippy, N.A., Dorenbos, K., Concepcion, R.C., Agarwal, A.K. and Rho, J.M. (2004) The ketogenic diet increases mitochondrial uncoupling protein levels and activity. *Ann Neurol* **55**, 576–580.

Szot, P., Weinshenker, D., Rho, J.M., Storey, T.W. and Schwartzkroin, P.A. (2001) Norepinephrine is required for the anticonvulsant effect of the ketogenic diet. *Brain Res Dev Brain Res* **129**, 211–214.

Thio, L.L., Wong, M. and Yamada, K.A. (2000) Ketone bodies do not directly alter excitatory or inhibitory hippocampal synaptic transmission. *Neurology* **54**, 325–331.

Thio, L.L., Erbayat-Altay, E., Rensing, N. and Yamada, K.A. (2006) Leptin contributes to slower weight gain in juvenile rodents on a ketogenic diet. *Pediatr Res* **60**, 413–417.

Uhlemann, E.R. and Neims, A.H. (1972) Anticonvulsant properties of the ketogenic diet in mice. *J Pharmacol Exp Ther* **180**, 231–238.

Wang, Z.J., Bergqvist, C., Hunter, J.V. et al. (2003) In vivo measurement of brain metabolites using two-dimensional double-quantum MR spectroscopy: exploration of GABA levels in a ketogenic diet. *Magn Reson Med* **49**, 615–619.

Willis, S., Stoll, J., Sweetman, L. and Borges, K. (2010) Anticonvulsant effects of a triheptanoin diet in two mouse chronic seizure models. *Neurobiol Dis* **40**, 565–572.

Wu, Z., Puigserver, P., Andersson, U. et al. (1999) Mechanisms controlling mitochondrial biogenesis and respiration through the thermogenic coactivator PGC-1. *Cell* **98**, 115–124.

Xu, L., Rensing, N., Yang, X.F. et al. (2008) Leptin inhibits 4-aminopyridine- and pentylenetetrazole-induced seizures and AMPAR-mediated synaptic transmission in rodents. *J Clin Invest* **118**, 272–280.

Yudkoff, M., Daikhin, Y., Horyn, O., Nissim, I. and Nissim, I. (2008) Ketosis and brain handling of glutamate, glutamine, and GABA. *Epilepsia* **49**, 73–75.

Section 2

Clinical Implementation

Chapter 6

Preparing for dietary treatment

Georgiana Fitzsimmons

UCL-Institute of Child Health and Great Ormond Street Hospital for
Children NHS Trust, London, UK

Ketogenic dietary therapy: the multidisciplinary team

Implementation of a ketogenic diet (KD) can be difficult and success depends on a number of core staff with a multidisciplinary team approach to the care of the child: a dietitian trained in the use of the KD, a neurologist or paediatrician with a special interest in epilepsy and experience of using the diet, and ideally a specialist nurse. This team must be able to advise and assist patients when they run into problems that are either caused or exacerbated by being on the diet. The support of a dietetic assistant, pharmacist and a clinical biochemist may also be useful for the core team.

Assessment of suitability for dietary treatment

Indications and contraindications for treatment with a KD are shown in Box 6.1. Consideration also needs to be given to the following problems.

- *Feeding difficulties.* KDs involve restricted dietary regimens and children with behavioural feeding difficulties should be identified and referred for appropriate treatment before being considered for dietary treatment, preferably referral to a behavioural feeding clinic (see Chapter 7).
- *Dysphagia and significant gastro-oesophageal reflux.* These need to be appropriately managed prior to starting a KD, and ideally should be addressed before the child is referred for dietary treatment. If the child has been under the care of a speech and language therapist because of dysphagia it is important that an up-to-date review has taken place before referral.
- *Enteral feeding.* If this is indicated, a gastrostomy needs to be inserted prior to starting a KD.

Dietary Treatment of Epilepsy: Practical Implementation of Ketogenic Therapy,
First Edition. Edited by Elizabeth Neal.

Box 6.1   Indications and contraindications for ketogenic dietary therapy.

Indications
Seizures fail to respond to two appropriate antiepileptic medications in therapeutic doses
Certain epilepsy syndromes early in their course:
Lennox–Gastaut syndrome
Myoclonic astatic epilepsy (Doose syndrome)
Dravet syndrome (severe myoclonic epilepsy of infancy)
Infantile spasms (West syndrome)
Symptomatic epilepsies if epilepsy surgery is not indicated, e.g. tuberous sclerosis, bilateral cortical malformations or diffuse bilateral brain injuries
Glucose transporter type 1 (GLUT-1) deficiency
Pyruvate dehydrogenase (PDH) deficiency
Intolerable and/or severe side effects from antiepileptic medications

Definite contraindications (see also Kossoff et al., 2009)
Fatty acid oxidation defects
Carnitine deficiencies
Organic acidurias
Pyruvate carboxylase deficiency
Familial hyperlipidaemia
Hypoglycaemia under investigation
Ketoneogenesis/ketolysis defects
Severe gastro-oesophageal reflux
Severe liver disease
Disorders requiring a high carbohydrate diet, e.g. acute intermittent porphyria
Non-compliance of patient or caregivers

Possible contraindications
Diabetes mellitus (medication adjustment may be required and careful monitoring essential)
Certain mitochondrial diseases (see also Kang et al., 2007; Lee et al., 2008)
Concomitant steroid use will limit ketosis

- *Dietary restrictions and food allergy.* Although these are not a contraindication to starting dietary treatment, multiple food allergies may make a KD inadvisable. Each child must be assessed on an individual basis by the dietitian.
- *Other.* KD therapy may not be suitable if the child has a history of renal stones or hyperlipidaemia or if taking diuretics or medications that increase the risk of acidosis. Suitability for treatment should be assessed by the paediatric neurologist.

Pre-diet evaluation

Before a diet is started an evaluation should be conducted by the KD team with the child and family. Following referral for KD therapy most centres in the UK invite families to attend a multidisciplinary clinic where the child's suitability for this treatment is assessed. This is also an opportunity to explain KD therapies

---

Box 6.2   Pre-diet dietetic nutritional assessment: factors to consider

- 3–4 day food record diary to assess current dietary intake, eating patterns and nutritional status
- Food preferences and restrictions
- Behavioural issues with food
- Food allergies or intolerances
- Swallowing difficulties
- Developmental feeding skills, food textures, thickened fluids
- Fluid intake and types
- Anthropometric measurements and recent growth trends (plot on centile charts to establish recent growth trends): weight, height/length (or alternative if not possible; see Chapter 18), head circumference (for children less than 2 years)
- Level of mobility and activity
- Vitamin and mineral supplements
- Bowel habits: frequency; foods, medications or nutritional products used to treat constipation

---

and possible side effects in detail, to take baseline laboratory tests and arrange any other medical investigations required. This section gives an outline of the information collected by each team member during the pre-diet evaluation interview with the family.

Dietetic assessment

It is essential for the dietitian to complete a comprehensive nutritional assessment before starting KD therapy (Box 6.2). This will help assess suitability for a dietary treatment, check a child's nutritional status, and give an indication of food preferences and eating patterns. This assessment can be used as the basis for deciding the most appropriate type of diet and for establishing dietary energy requirements and developing suitable meal plans. A suggested proforma for baseline dietetic assessment is shown in the Supplement to this chapter.

Neurological and epilepsy evaluation by a paediatric neurologist

Children referred for KD therapy should be under the care of a neurologist or a paediatrician with a special interest in epilepsy. The consultant overseeing the dietary treatment should be readily available to support and advise other members of the team when families run into problems either caused or exacerbated by being on the diet. A thorough pre-diet neurological assessment is essential (Box 6.3), and throughout dietary treatment the patient should be seen and reviewed regularly by the neurologist. In the UK most teams see children regularly in a multidisciplinary clinic to assess progress on the diet, for example 3 and 6 months after starting the diet, and then every 6 months. Children may be seen more frequently as clinically indicated.

Box 6.3   Pre-diet neurological assessment: factors to consider

The underlying diagnosis
- Is it epilepsy?
- Type of epilepsy (see Chapter 2)

Is dietary treatment appropriate?
- Indications and contraindications (see Box 6.1)
- Epilepsy optimally treated to date?
- Current and past antiepileptic medications optimal?
- Suitable for surgical consideration or other non-pharmacological treatment options? (see Chapter 3)

Child and family expectations from the diet: are these achievable?
- Seizure control
- Reduction in antiepileptic medications
- Improvement in life quality
- Individual goals

Seizure assessment for monitoring
- Type
- Frequency

General
- Associated illnesses or conditions
- General paediatric and neurological examination
- Developmental progress
- Education

Clinical nurse specialist assessment and education

Ideally the multidisciplinary team should include a clinical nurse specialist with training in epilepsy. The clinical nurse specialist plays an important role in educating the family about ketone and seizure monitoring and illness management, and can be a useful liaison between the local services, for example schools, family doctors and local hospitals, and can assist in educating these agencies about the diet (Box 6.4).

The dietetic assistant

A dietetic assistant is a very useful member of a KD team and can support the dietitian by assisting with analysis of food records, collating written material for parent teaching sessions, arranging prescriptions for nutritional products, and registering families for home deliveries of products. Having this extra support allows more dietetic time to focus on establishing children on the diet and providing follow-up and support to those already on the diet.

Box 6.4   Pre-diet: the role of the clinical nurse specialist

Baseline laboratory and medical investigations
- Provide necessary documentation for families
- Ensure baseline laboratory tests completed and reviewed by doctor prior to starting treatment

Medications
- Check formulations and change if necessary (in liaison with neurologist) to minimize carbohydrate content in antiepileptic and other medications
- Arrange prescriptions for medications added to prevent side effects of the diet (laxatives, medications to prevent renal stones)

Education
- Ketone and seizure monitoring
- Guidelines for use during intercurrent illness or medical treatment for health professionals and families

Liaison
- Pharmacies: arrange and advise on prescriptions for alternative lower carbohydrate preparations
- Family doctor and local paediatric team
- Schools and nurseries

Box 6.5   Medical investigations which may be required pre-diet

- *Renal ultrasound scan*: for children under 2 years old, and children on topiramate, zonisamide or acetazolamide, or who have a family history of renal calculi
- *Video telemetry*: if non-epileptogenic attacks are suspected or to delineate the seizure type if required
- *Electrocardiogram (ECG)*: if evidence of cardiomyopathy or hypertension
- *Electroencephalogram (EEG) (awake and sleep)*: if last recording more than 6 months ago
- *Cerebrospinal fluid*: glucose level if GLUT-1 deficiency suspected
- *Dual-energy X-ray absorptiometry (DEXA) scan*: if a child stays on the diet there may be a risk of developing osteopenia (see Chapter 19). In the UK some centres are currently monitoring bone density scans annually and collecting serial data for children who stay on the diet for longer than 3 months

Pre-diet laboratory tests and medical investigations

Before starting children on a dietary treatment certain laboratory tests (see Chapter 18) and medical investigations are required (Box 6.5). Although each centre will have their own protocol for baseline evaluations and monitoring, most guidelines are similar. The results of urinary organic acid test, and any other metabolic tests pending, should be reviewed prior to initiation of dietary treatment to ensure the child does not have a metabolic disorder that would contraindicate the use of a high-fat low-carbohydrate diet. These investigations may have already been completed as part of the work-up to determine an epilepsy diagnosis. Metabolic investigations may take time to be analysed so it is important they are completed early in the course of evaluating a child's suitability for dietary treatment.

Preparing families for dietary treatment

It is important to ensure that patients, families and carers are fully informed about the dietary treatment that they hope to start (Box 6.6). When assessing a child's suitability for KD therapy, the team should establish with the patient and family *realistic* expectations of the dietary treatment. The goals that the patients and parents hope to achieve should be agreed and documented before proceeding with the treatment. An initial 3-month trial of a KD is usually recommended and these goals should be reviewed at follow-up appointments; they may be helpful in making decisions with the family about continuing with the diet.

Box 6.6   Additional factors to discuss with families in pre-diet multidisciplinary clinic

Rationale and evidence for the dietary treatments

Agree and document desired/acceptable outcome and goals

Implications of the diets
- Restricted low-carbohydrate, high-fat diet
- Some versions of the diet require food to be weighed
- Regular monitoring required: liaison with dietitians, measurements of ketones, seizures, weight, and clinic visits
- Side effects of the diet (provide reassurance that these may be avoided or alleviated by manipulation of the diet)

Time frames for treatment
- Initial 3-month trial
- Epilepsy: treatment for up to 2 years if beneficial. Some centres wean the diet after 2 years to evaluate the benefits of the diet for the child
- At each clinic visit discuss the impact for the child and family and how difficult it is for them to continue on the diet
- GLUT-1 and PDH deficiency: the diet may be continued until adolescence for these patients but requires assessment on an individual basis

Expected time frame for the diet to take effect

Monitoring the diet
- Baseline laboratory investigations required and frequency
- Measuring ketosis
- Other medical investigations may also be required

Commitment to the treatment required from all those involved in the child's care

---

Deciding which dietary treatment to use

Palatability and ease of use for the family and child need to be taken into account when choosing which type of diet to use. A food diary, kept for 3 or 4 days, should be the basis for the type of diet chosen. Family preference should also be taken into account. Table 6.1 discusses some of the pros and cons of each diet type and Table 6.2 lists some of the factors to consider when choosing the most appropriate diet for a child. These are guidelines only and each patient needs to be assessed on an individual basis. It is possible to change from one diet to another if the initial type of diet is unsuitable (see Chapter 21).

Advice on pre-diet meal manipulation

There is evidence to suggest a pre-diet manipulation of meals may lead to better adaptation to, and acceptance of, a KD at initiation (Rizzutti et al., 2007). Most centres will provide pre-diet information to patients on waiting lists for dietary

Table 6.1   Pros and cons of different types of ketogenic dietary therapies.

Diet type	Pros	Cons
Classical ketogenic diet	More experience in use of classical diet and more widely used Most suitable choice for tube feeds Strict prescription	Meals appear small because of high-fat content Very restricted carbohydrate and protein
Medium-chain triglyceride (MCT) ketogenic diet	Less fat allows inclusion of more protein and carbohydrate and a more varied diet	MCT may cause gastrointestinal side effects or cause a laxative effect, especially in larger doses MCT must be taken with every meal/snack
Modified Atkin's diet (MAD)	Free protein and calories No need to weigh foods May help families or teenagers who might otherwise find more restrictive diets too difficult	Still requires generous amount of fat Carbohydrate very restricted at 10–20 g/day May be difficult longer term to keep tight control on calories May require more parent/carer input in designing meals/managing diet
Low glycaemic index treatment (LGIT)	More generous carbohydrate allowance Low glycaemic index carbohydrates may have other health benefits Household measures used rather than food weighing	May require more parent/carer input in designing meals/managing diet Carbohydrate allowance includes fibre so may seem less in practice

Table 6.2   Deciding which diet to use: considerations.

Factors to consider	Dietary treatment
Age under 2 years	Classical KD may be most suitable as more structured meal plans can be given. Very high fat meals are smaller and may be easier for the child to complete. MAD not recommended
Age over 2 years	Either classical, MCT or MAD may be suitable
Older children and teenagers	MCT, MAD or LGIT
Food preferences	High intakes of carbohydrate pre-diet or picky eaters may do better with MCT diet as less carbohydrate restriction is required. Consider the child's ability to consistently take MCT supplement
Nutritional assessment	MAD or LGIT may be less suitable if considered at nutritional risk
Children with nasogastric or gastrostomy tubes, infants on formula as a sole source of nutrition	The classical diet is the preferred option for these children as there is a complete powdered formula available (see Chapters 14 and 22)

Box 6.7   Possible adjustments to usual meals before starting dietary treatment

- Increase fat intake by using full fat products rather than low-fat, e.g. milk, yoghurts and spreads
- Decrease refined carbohydrate intake, e.g. avoid adding sugar to foods and drinks, change to sugar free squashes and diet fizzy drinks
- Establish regular meal and snack times
- Encourage all offered meals and snacks to be eaten

---

treatment. This would usually include the principles of the diet and suggested alterations to intake which will help acclimatize the patient to the prospective change in fat and carbohydrate intake (Box 6.7). This also allows patients and families to make an informed choice regarding a therapeutic diet as a treatment option and may help reduce dietetic time used calculating meals for those who cannot or will not tolerate meals on a restrictive diet. It is important that pre-diet manipulation is initiated only when a provisional start date is pending, and after discussion with the dietitian. Extended periods of pre-diet manipulation and carbohydrate restriction could be harmful, and lead to hypoglycaemia, hyperketosis, excess weight gain or weight loss. It may not be appropriate to restrict pre-diet carbohydrate intake for children with glucose transporter type 1 deficiency, pyruvate dehydrogenase deficiency or mitochondrial disorders.

Some families will want to start shopping for suitable ingredients before their child starts on a dietary treatment. There are some essential items and ingredients required for smooth initiation of these diets (see Chapter 13).

Summary

Preparing for a dietary treatment will include an assessment for suitability and a pre-diet evaluation, ideally by a multidisciplinary team. This will include both nutritional and neurological assessment, laboratory tests and medical investigations. Discussion must also include choosing the most appropriate type of KD therapy and establishing realistic outcome expectations.

Acknowledgements

This chapter is based in part on the Great Ormond Street Hospital Clinical Guidelines for the Ketogenic Diet 2010 by C. Eltze, G.J. Fitzsimmons, M. Sewell and H.M. Chaffe.

References

Kang, H.C., Lee, Y.M., Kim, H.D., Lee, J.S. and Slama, A. (2007) Safe and effective use of the ketogenic diet in children with epilepsy and mitochondrial respiratory chain complex defects. *Epilepsia* **48**, 82–88.

Kossoff, E.H., Zupec-Kania, B.A., Amark, P.E. et al. (2009) Optimal clinical management of children receiving the ketogenic diet: recommendations of the International Ketogenic Diet Study Group. *Epilepsia* **50**, 304–317.

Lee, Y.M., Kang, H.C., Lee, J.S. et al. (2008) Mitochondrial respiratory chain defects: underlying etiology in various epileptic conditions. *Epilepsia* **49**, 685–690.

Rizzutti, S., Ramos, A.M.F., Muszkat, M. and Gabbai, A.A. (2007) Is hospitalisation really necessary during the introduction of the ketogenic diet? *J Child Neurol* **22**, 33–37.

Shaw, V. and Lawson, M. (eds) (2007) *Clinical Paediatric Dietetics*, 3rd edn. Oxford: Blackwell Publishing Ltd.

Supplement to chapter

Suggested proforma for baseline dietetic assessment before commencing ketogenic dietary therapy (adapted from Shaw and Lawson, 2007).

Name:				
Date of birth:				
Hospital number:				
Date:				
Weight:	kg		Centile	
Height:	cm		Centile	
Consistency of food:	Normal	Soft	Puree	Fluid
Types of fluids:			Daily volume:	
Consistency of fluids:	Normal	Syrup	Custard	
	Thickener used:		Quantity:	
Reason(s)	Dysphagia	Regurgitation	GO reflux	
Frequency of defecation:	Times per day		Times per week	
	Pain	Bleeding per rectum	Stool consistency	
Laxative use (preparation and dosage):	Lactulose: Movicol Paediatric: Sodium picosulphate: Senna: Resource Optifibre: Other:			

Typical meal pattern:

Breakfast	
Snack	
Lunch	
Snack	
Evening meal	
Bedtime snack	
Time taken over an average meal:	Percent eaten of food offered:
Gastrostomy/other feeding tube *in situ*:	

Nutrient-dense/energy-dense supplement(s)/ gastrostomy feeds:	Name of preparation(s), dose:		Frequency	
Other supplement(s): preparation and dosage	Iron Zinc Calcium ± vitamin D$_3$ Carnitine Selenium Other vitamins Other			
Mobility:				
Activities:				
Others involved in care:	Respite	Nursery	School	
Current medications	Name	Dose	Formulation	Carbohydrate content
Previous medications tried:				
Seizures	Types:		Frequency:	
Sleep patterns:				
Baseline blood and urine investigations completed and reviewed by team				
Child and family's expectations from the dietary treatment				
Approximate daily intake from 3-day food record:				
Protein in g (convert to g/kg)		Normal DRV* in g (convert to g/kg)		
Energy in kcal (convert to kcal/kg)		Normal DRV* in kcal (convert to kcal/kg)		
Estimated requirements for ketogenic dietary therapy				
Protein in g (convert to g/kg)				
Energy in kcal (convert to kcal/kg)				
Comments/action				

*DRV, dietary reference value for age and gender-matched healthy child.

Chapter 7

The challenge of therapeutic diets in children with pre-existing feeding problems

Bridget Lambert[1] and Mary-Anne Leung[2]

[1]*Vitaflo International Ltd, Liverpool, UK*
[2]*Evelina Children's Hospital, London, UK*

Ketogenic diet (KD) therapies are restrictive and challenging regimens and a high degree of compliance is necessary. Many children referred for these dietary treatments will already have pre-existing feeding problems, which may be physical or behavioural, or both. Ideally, feeding difficulties likely to compromise food intake should be identified and resolved before starting treatment so as not to add to the burden of undertaking these diets. However, their pre-existence does not necessarily preclude trying a diet and experiencing success in the longer term. For example, some children with physical feeding difficulties find the reduced size of meals due to their high fat and energy content means eating is quicker and more enjoyable. Likewise, children who self-restrict their food choices may be very accepting of the necessary dietary restrictions and be content to have the same meals and snacks every day. This chapter focuses on the types of feeding problems frequently seen in children referred for a KD therapy.

Physical feeding difficulties

Oral motor impairment and swallowing dysfunction are commonly associated with neurological disability, frequently occurring in children with cerebral palsy and neurodegenerative conditions such as Rett syndrome and brain tumours. In addition to interfering with the process of eating and drinking, the risk of aspiration is increased and feeding times can be prolonged. Nutritional intake can be compromised leading to malnutrition particularly in those most severely affected. Symptoms resulting from foregut dysmotility, gastro-oesophageal reflux, delayed

Dietary Treatment of Epilepsy: Practical Implementation of Ketogenic Therapy,
First Edition. Edited by Elizabeth Neal.
© 2012 John Wiley & Sons, Ltd. Published 2012 by John Wiley & Sons, Ltd.

gastric emptying and constipation related to the neurological defect can also negatively affect feeding success and enjoyment. Carers can spend many hours preparing food and feeding their child, and the process can be a source of much distress and anxiety to them (Sullivan et al., 2000, 2002; Sullivan, 2008).

The estimated prevalence of epilepsy in children with cerebral palsy is 30% and in paediatric neurological disorders as a whole between 25 and 35% (Braathen and Theorell, 1995; Sullivan et al., 2000; Singhi et al., 2003; Berg et al., 2008). Essentially, the risk of epilepsy rises with severity of motor disorder and intellectual disability. Of these children, a proportion will have feeding problems significant enough to require medical or surgical intervention, such as medication, the insertion of a gastrostomy and/or an anti-reflux procedure (fundoplication). The prevalence of epilepsy is higher in children attending specialist feeding clinics for severe gastrointestinal and feeding problems; estimates range from 47% (Venkasteswaran and Shevell, 2008) to 60% (Somerville et al., 2008).

If a child with epilepsy and known physical feeding problems is referred for a dietary treatment for epilepsy it is important to have up-to-date and relevant clinical information about the difficulties the child is experiencing and any current therapy or interventions being given. Parents and/or carers should be thoroughly consulted about their child's feeding problems to establish how they try to manage them and to find out about any specific issues and concerns they may have about their child's ability to eat and drink. An accurate assessment of current dietary intake should be made. Direct observation of the child being fed and given a drink can be very useful. All these details will aid in the decision-making process regarding the appropriateness of the KD therapy for the child as an individual and for their carers who will be carrying it out at home.

The following points should be considered when planning and instituting a KD therapy.

- For a child with pre-existing gastro-oesophageal reflux and constipation, a high-fat diet may aggravate symptoms further as gastric emptying is delayed and gut transit time slowed. If the child is not already on treatment such as laxatives or anti-reflux medication, these may become necessary once on the diet. Carers should be aware of this and seek medical advice as appropriate. In particular, maintaining a regular bowel habit is vital as constipation can increase seizure activity and impact on any benefit of the diet.
- If there are concerns about aspiration or swallowing difficulties, investigations such as a pH study or videofluoroscopy and any necessary interventions should be performed pre-diet.
- If the child is already receiving input from a speech and language therapist, occupational therapist or physiotherapist, their professional assessment of feeding ability is essential in order to make certain safe and effective feeding techniques are being followed. Future follow-up should continue with these professionals once the diet is started or children should be referred to these services as indicated.

- School, community and respite nurses involved in the care of the child are invaluable sources of contact, and can help in the practical management of issues such as enteral feeding, constipation, weighing and measuring.
- If the child is already under the care of a local dietitian, liaison is vital, particularly for background information on feeding ability, growth history and current feed and/or dietary intake. They may be willing to share care and assist with follow-up, for example monitoring weight and height, troubleshooting enteral feeding problems and organizing supplies of feed and associated equipment.
- Some children with feeding difficulties lose food and fluid from their mouth whilst eating or drinking which is not replaced. Information should be obtained about spillages and these should be taken into account when estimating energy intake before calculating the diet.
- The texture and consistency of foods and fluids usually eaten and managed by the child should be noted to ensure appropriate meals and snacks are calculated and prescribed. Some children may choke on lumps or on foods that require biting or chewing, making them unsafe to eat and swallow. However, the high fat content of the KD therapy means meals are generally soft and hence very suitable for those that require mashed or pureed foods.
- Adequate hydration can be a problem for children with oro-motor impairment due to difficulties with controlling liquid in their mouth or losses from drooling saliva. Fluid intake should be determined, optimized before starting KD therapy and then monitored once on a diet to help prevent side effects such as constipation and acidosis. If there is a risk of aspiration and the child requires a fluid thickener, a carbohydrate-free one should be used.
- A number of children with severe feeding problems have a gastrostomy. The KD can be given as an enteral feed (see Chapter 14).

Growth and energy requirements

Regular growth monitoring is recommended while on a KD therapy to ensure an appropriate dietary energy prescription (see Chapter 18); however, children with neurological impairment can be growth restricted prior to starting a prescribed diet. They have different growth patterns from their unaffected peers which are not taken into account by normal centile charts. Although these can be used if results are interpreted with care, centile charts for cerebral palsy are available (Day et al., 2007) that account for not just age but also level of disability (available at www.LifeExpectancy.org/articles/GrowthCharts.shtml). Specialized equipment may be required for the child to be weighed safely and this can usually be carried out at school or a respite facility on request. Reliable measurements of height or length can be more difficult to obtain in disabled children due to postural constraints or contractures but equations that estimate height from limb lengths are available (Stevenson, 1995).

Depending on mobility, energy requirements for children with neurological disabilities and physical feeding problems may be well below those expected for their age. Although there are a variety of calculations that can be used to estimate these, in practice obtaining a detailed dietary and growth history prior to starting the diet, then regular monitoring of growth plus analysis and refinement of nutritional intake once it is established will determine individual energy needs just as adequately (Lambert and Han, 2009). If the diet is successful, dietary energy requirements may increase or decrease due to changes in activity levels and the diet prescription will need altering; an adequate protein intake should always be maintained (see Chapter 17).

Behavioural feeding difficulties

Behavioural feeding difficulties are very common in children and mild feeding problems have been reported in 25–35 % of normal children (Rudolph, 2002). In a community study of parents of infants and toddlers, 62 % reported more than one feeding concern (Reau et al., 1996). Feeding difficulties tend to fall into three main categories.

- Problem with quantity: disinterest, food avoidance, poor appetite.
- Problem with range: selective and faddy eaters.
- Problem with texture: inappropriate food texture for age.

Very often a child who has feeding problems has experienced a history of physically unpleasant sensations associated with feeding, such as vomiting with gastro-oesophageal reflux, structural defects of the oropharynx and gastric motility problems, and this learnt association creates food avoidance and refusal. Food refusal is stressful for parents and sometimes they can unwittingly reinforce food refusal behaviour in their child. It is not uncommon if a child refuses to eat a non-preferred food for the parents to eventually give up and then offer the preferred food.

Behavioural feeding problems do not always negate a child commencing a KD therapy and it is possible for the dietitian to plan a diet that is acceptable (Box 7.1). However, it may be useful to try some particular strategies to help the feeding difficulties prior to starting a prescribed diet (Box 7.2). The skill of the dietitian is to discuss which strategies will be helpful for an individual child, as what will work for one child will not work for another. It is very important that the child and family are given goals that they can achieve as success gives confidence.

Feeding problems and autistic spectrum disorder

Children with autistic spectrum disorder (ASD) commonly have feeding problems and this has been reported to be as high as 90 % (Kodak and Piazza, 2008; Volkert and Vaz, 2010). The diet can be restricted to a very few foods and 70 %

Box 7.1   Case report of using the KD in a child with behavioural feeding problems

Presentation
- Girl of 6 years
- Diagnosis of Dravet syndrome
- Learning difficulties and severe attention deficit hyperactivity disorder
- Referral for assessment of a KD. Parents had recently attended a Dravet conference and were very keen to trial the diet as their daughter had a prescription of four antiepileptic medications

Normal diet
- Breakfast: hot chocolate, small pot of fromage frais
- Mid morning: cubes of cheddar cheese, occasional crisps and fruit juice
- School lunch: potato or pasta, cheese or fish, various vegetables, fruit and custard or ice cream
- Mid afternoon: cheese, fruit and fruit juice
- Dinner: salmon or sausage or houmous or scrambled egg, avocado with olive oil and cream cheese, yoghurt. Each evening meal had to be served with 40 g cubed cheddar cheese
- Drinks: water, fruit juice and hot chocolate

At home, meals were often stressful and the diet restricted. She would not eat potato, rice or bread, but would eat lumps of butter. At school a wide range of foods were eaten.

Dietetic assessment and plan
The classical KD was suitable for this child as there was already a preference for some high-fat foods. It was important that the portion of cheddar cheese at dinner be incorporated into the meal plan. A 3:1 ratio was used and the prescribed daily diet divided into three meals and two snacks. Several recipes were provided for each meal. The dinner recipes included some cheddar cheese that could be cubed. A prescribed vitamin and mineral supplement (Phlexy-vits, Nutricia) was included.

Example KD meal plan
- Breakfast: Ketocal (Nutricia) milk shake, light yoghurt with double cream
- Lunch: packed lunch for school, e.g. vegetable omelette, houmous with mayonnaise and cucumber, salmon and vegetables in a creamy sauce
- Dinner: scrambled egg or omelette with cheddar cheese, avocado and olive oil with cheddar cheese
- Snacks: Ketocal smoothie or milk shake, Ketocal cheese crackers, houmous with mayonnaise and cucumber sticks

Post starting dietary treatment
During the first 3 months the child had moderate ketosis; intercurrent illnesses may have prevented higher levels being achieved. The KD was accepted by the child, although it is still too early to predict if the diet is helping to control seizures.

---

of these children have been described as selective eaters (Twachtman-Reilly et al., 2008; Volkert and Vaz, 2010). These children are often very sensitive to the smell, texture and presentation of food. Mixed textures and lumps are frequently avoided. Children with ASD often like foods to be predictable and can reject foods if the packaging changes. Fruit and vegetables are not predictable as they

Box 7.2 Management of behavioural feeding difficulties prior to starting dietary treatment

- Encourage regular meals and snacks. Some meal time rearrangement may be helpful if there are long gaps between meals or the child is too tired to eat.
- Limit the time for meals to about 20 minutes.
- Avoid force feeding as this will not motivate a child to eat more food. It is distressing for both child and parents and meal times will become fearful and dreaded.
- Offer small energy-dense portions of food. Small quantities of different foods presented separately are often better accepted than large portions.
- Offer smooth purée and then finger 'bite and dissolve' type foods as many children dislike mixed textures which can cause gagging. Avoid mixed textures such as meat and vegetables in sauce.
- Encourage children in the preparation for meals when possible by shopping for food and helping to set the table and prepare the food.
- Reward stickers are helpful in the very short term for some children. However, more success may be achieved if children are encouraged to keep scrap activity books of foods that they do eat.
- Avoid all negative talk around a child not eating. Children respond well to praise and non-food rewards such a story or special toy.
- Encourage a child to eat with the family rather than alone. Peer modelling often influences a child to eat.

Box 7.3 Further strategies for management of feeding problems in ASD

- A programme devised by a specialist feeding team to desensitize a child to a food by firstly touching a food, then smelling, then licking and then finally tasting a food.
- Gradually widening the intake of accepted foods, e.g. a sweet biscuit to a semi-sweet biscuit and then to a savoury cracker.
- For some children 'social stories' are helpful in improving their feeding behaviour and a specialist speech and language therapist can help with writing a suitable story for each individual.
- Vitamin and mineral supplements may be recommended for children on restricted diets. It is often more successful if they are given as a medicine away from meals; perhaps the child can syringe the supplement for themselves. Mixing supplements into food can lead to further problems as the child can then become suspicious of all foods.

can vary in colour and texture and this is why they are so often refused. The environment can be important for some children and it is not uncommon for them to eat a particular food in one place and not another. Some of the interventions already recommended may work but quite often these children need to be assessed and managed by a specialist feeding team and need further strategies (Box 7.3). A dietitian working with children with ASD needs to be creative, practical and to have realistic expectations. A perfect diet may not be achieved but an improved diet should be possible.

Summary

A significant proportion of children referred for a dietary treatment for their epilepsy will already have physical or behavioural feeding difficulties. These will present additional challenges and should be identified and treated prior to starting a prescribed diet. With appropriate management most children can be successfully initiated and maintained on a KD therapy.

References

Berg, A.T., Langfitt, J.T., Testa, F.M. et al. (2008) Global cognitive function in children with epilepsy: a community-based study. *Epilepsia* **49**, 608–614.

Braathen, G. and Theorell, K. (1995) A general hospital population of childhood epilepsy. *Acta Paediatr* **84**, 1143–1146.

Day, S.M., Strauss, D.J., Vachon, P.J., Rosenbloom, L., Sharvelle, R.M. and Wu, Y.W. (2007) Growth patterns in a population of children and adolescents with cerebral palsy. *Dev Med Child Neurol* **49**, 167–171.

Kodak, T. and Piazza, C.C. (2008) Assessment and behavioral treatment of feeding and sleeping disorders in children with autism spectrum disorders. *Child Adolesc Psychiatr Clin North Am* **17**, 887–905.

Lambert, B.R. and Han, W.M. (2009) Feeding and dietetic assessment and management. In: Sullivan, P.B. (ed.) *Feeding and Nutrition in Children with Neurodevelopmental Disability*. London: McKeith Press, pp. 57–85.

Reau, N.R., Senturia, Y.D., Lebailly, S.A. and Christoffel, K.K. (1996) Infant and toddler feeding patterns and problems: normative data and a new direction. *J Dev Behav Pediatr* **17**, 149–153.

Rudolph, C.D. (2002) Feeding disorders in infants and children. *Pediatr Clin North Am* **49**, 97–112.

Singhi, P., Jagirdar, S., Khandelwal, N. and Malhi, P. (2003) Epilepsy in children with cerebral palsy. *J Child Neurol* **18**, 174–179.

Somerville, H., Tzannes, G., Wood, J. et al. (2008) Gastrointestinal and nutritional problems in severe developmental disability. *Dev Med Child Neurol* **50**, 712–716.

Stevenson, R.D. (1995) Use of segmental measures to estimate stature in children with cerebral palsy. *Arch Pediatr Adolesc Med* **149**, 658–662.

Sullivan, P.B. (2008) Gastrointestinal disorders in children with neurodevelopmental disabilities. *Dev Disabil Res Rev* **14**, 128–136.

Sullivan, P.B., Lambert, B., Rose, M., Ford-Adams, M., Johnson, M.A. and Griffiths, P. (2000) Prevalence and severity of feeding and nutritional problems in children with neurological impairment: Oxford Feeding Study. *Dev Med Child Neurol* **42**, 674–680.

Sullivan, P.B., Juszczak, E., Lambert, B.R., Rose, M., Ford-Adams, M.E. and Johnson, A. (2002) Impact of feeding problems on nutritional intake and growth: Oxford Feeding Study II. *Dev Med Child Neurol* **44**, 461–467.

Twachtman-Reilly, J., Amaral, S.C. and Zebrowski, P.P. (2008) Addressing feeding disorders in children on the autism spectrum in school-based settings: physiological and behavioral issues. *Language, Speech and Hearing Services in Schools* **39**, 261–272.

Venkateswaran, S. and Shevell, M.I. (2008) Co-morbidities and clinical determinants of outcome in children with spastic quadriplegic cerebral palsy. *Dev Med Child Neurol* **50**, 216–222.

Volkert, V.M. and Vaz, P.C. (2010) Recent studies on feeding problems in children with autism. *J Appl Behav Anal* **43**, 155–159.

Chapter 8

The classical ketogenic diet

Gwyneth Magrath and Elizabeth Neal

Matthew's Friends Charity and Clinics, Lingfield, UK

The classical ketogenic diet (KD) was first described in early studies (see Chapter 1) and the basic principles for calculating a dietary prescription remain very similar today. This chapter explains how to calculate a classical KD prescription, and then use this to develop meals by calculating recipes. An alternative exchange system approach is also included.

The energy prescription

The energy prescription for a KD should be sufficient to allow normal growth and development whilst on the diet, at the same time maintaining the level of ketosis needed for optimal efficacy. Excess dietary energy and weight gain will cause poor ketosis, which can in turn compromise potential seizure control. A comprehensive individual pre-diet nutritional assessment is necessary (see Chapter 6), including a food record diary from which normal pre-KD energy intake can be calculated. Anthropometric measurements will also have been performed, and recent growth trends should be reviewed. A rough assessment of energy expenditure can be made based on mobility, level of physical activity, anticonvulsant medication usage and seizure activity. Energy expenditure is unlikely to be at normal levels for age for a child who is having multiple seizures; their usual children's activities will probably be curtailed. Anticonvulsant medication may also make them lethargic and drowsy. In some cases the child may be wheelchair bound. As well as reducing physical activity, the seizures and medication may also interfere with their ability to eat sufficient to maintain adequate nutrition. The initial KD energy prescription therefore takes into account the following criteria for each individual patient.

- Age.
- Current weight and height and recent growth trends.

Dietary Treatment of Epilepsy: Practical Implementation of Ketogenic Therapy,
First Edition. Edited by Elizabeth Neal.
© 2012 John Wiley & Sons, Ltd. Published 2012 by John Wiley & Sons, Ltd.

- Energy expenditure based on mobility, level of physical activity, and seizure activity.
- Medication use.
- Individual pre-KD energy intake.
- Estimated average requirement for energy intake (EAR) for age (this is a UK recommendation; Department of Health, 1991).

Some KD recommendations suggest a moderate dietary energy restriction is of benefit to ketosis and seizure control, although each child should be individually assessed as above. The following guidelines are recommended.

- If weight and height are on the correct centile for age and the child is capable of reasonable physical activity, the energy prescription should start with a 10–15% reduction of EAR appropriate to the child's age. A good start point could be to calculate 80–90% of EAR, then use an average between this and the pre-KD daily energy intake.
- When the weight is on a centile for age lower than the corresponding height centile it is prudent initially to allow the EAR for age. This is particularly important if recent growth trends show a child's weight to be tracking down the centiles. It is unlikely that the pre-KD energy intake will have been adequate; this should be evident from the diet history. This energy level may need adjustment later if the necessary ketosis is not achieved.
- When the child is wheelchair bound and on the correct centiles for height and weight, pre-KD energy intake is likely to be less than the EAR for age. In these cases the KD energy prescription should remain low with an up to 20% reduction in the EAR for age; this should at least not exceed the child's normal pre-KD energy intake. However, if the child's former intake was very low and he or she is underweight, even if mobility is restricted, the KD energy prescription should be less restricted: a 10% reduction in EAR would be enough initially.

An initial dietary energy prescription will need to be closely monitored and adjusted as needed, especially during the first few weeks and months of treatment. If the prescribed energy intake does not maintain growth it must be increased, and likewise if weight gain is excessive it will lead to poor ketosis and energy will need to be reduced. Dietary energy increases and decreases should always be done in controlled increments (see Chapter 17).

The protein prescription

In 1927 Talbot and colleagues concluded from their studies that a KD providing 1 g per kilogram of expected body weight would maintain nitrogen equilibrium and allow a small protein quota for growth; a positive nitrogen balance was achieved on this low protein intake in nearly all their 12 reported cases, who ranged from 2 to 22 years of age (Talbot et al., 1927). Classical KD guidelines usually suggest a

Table 8.1   Safe levels of protein intake for weaned infants, children up to 10 years (both sexes) and adolescent boys and girls. From World Health Organization (2007).

Age (years)	Safe level of protein intake (g per kg body weight)		
	Both sexes	**Girls**	**Boys**
0.5	1.31		
1	1.14		
1.5	1.03		
2	0.97		
3	0.90		
4	0.86		
5	0.85		
6	0.89		
7	0.91		
8	0.92		
9	0.92		
10	0.91		
11		0.90	0.91
12		0.89	0.90
13		0.88	0.90
14		0.87	0.89
15		0.85	0.88
16		0.84	0.87
17		0.83	0.86
18		0.82	0.85

prescription of 1–1.5 g of protein per kilogram body weight according to age, the rapidly growing younger child requiring the higher amount; this may be lower in adolescents (Freeman et al., 2007; Neal and Magrath, 2007). Recommendations for safe levels of protein requirements can be found in the latest World Health Organization (2007) technical report on this subject, summarized in Table 8.1. The amount of protein allowed in a classical KD prescription will usually include that provided from all types of food but protein quality must also be considered due to the importance of meeting requirements of all indispensable amino acids. The allowed amount of protein will be in many cases only just above the recommended safe levels, so high biological value sources should be chosen wherever possible. This point cannot be emphasized too strongly when using the classical KD.

The diet ratio

The classical KD is calculated using the ratio method that was first described over 80 years ago (Talbot et al., 1927; Talbot, 1930). A ketogenic ratio tells us the proportion (in grams) of fat in the diet as compared with carbohydrate and protein, for example a typical 4 : 1 ratio refers to a diet with a ratio of 4 g of fat to 1 g of protein plus carbohydrate combined. The diet is usually started at a lower

Table 8.2 Explanation of the ratio system used to calculate the classical KD.

Diet ratio	Macronutrient proportions		Percentage of dietary energy from macronutrients	
	Fat (g)	Protein and carbohydrate combined (g)	Fat (%)	Protein and carbohydrate combined (%)
1:1	1	1	69	31
2:1	2	1	82	18
3:1	3	1	87	13
4:1	4	1	90	10
5:1	5	1	92	8

ratio, such as 2:1, which can then be slowly increased until ketosis is achieved. Not every child will need the ratio of 4:1 to produce adequate ketosis to control their seizures. Table 8.2 gives more detail on KD ratios.

Diet prescription

Having decided upon the required energy, protein and ratio, the diet is calculated to give the prescribed daily amounts of fat, protein and carbohydrate. The easiest method is by using dietary units. A dietary unit is calculated from the calorie content of each of the macronutrients in the chosen diet ratio, based on fat providing 9 kcal/g and protein and carbohydrate providing 4 kcal/g each (kcal = kilocalorie of energy). This is explained clearly with worked examples in the excellent KD book by Kossoff et al. (2011) from Johns Hopkins Hospital, Baltimore, USA. Their method is widely employed throughout the world and is shown in Box 8.1 for the 4:1, 3:1 and 2:1 ratios.

The total daily dietary energy allowance is then divided by the kcal per dietary unit (this will depend on which ratio is to be chosen, for example if a 4:1 ratio, then the total energy will be divided by 40). This gives the number of dietary units that are allowed daily. This number is then multiplied by the units of fat in the ratio to give the total daily allowance of fat. The units of carbohydrate and protein in the ratio is 1, and this is multiplied by the number of allowed daily dietary units to give the total daily amount of both macronutrients together. The protein allowance has already been determined; this can then be subtracted to give the amount of carbohydrate. Once the daily amounts of fat, protein and carbohydrate have been calculated, they can be equally divided into three or four meals as required. If snacks are added to the daily menu, they must be taken from the overall daily prescription. All meals and snacks must be in the same diet ratio and therefore the relative proportions of fat, carbohydrate and protein must remain the same. For example, if a meal with a 4:1 ratio has 32 g of fat, 4 g of protein and 4 g of carbohydrate, then a snack with the same ratio providing 1 g of protein would have 8 g of fat and 1 g of carbohydrate. All diets will require an additional vitamin, mineral and trace element supplement (see Chapter 12). An example calculation is shown in Box 8.2.

Box 8.1   Diet prescription

Ratio 4:1
Each dietary unit = 4 g fat and 1 g protein and carbohydrate
Energy content of each dietary unit = (4 × 9 kcal) + (1 × 4 kcal) = 40 kcal

Ratio 3:1
Each dietary unit = 3 g fat and 1 g protein and carbohydrate
Energy content of each dietary unit = (3 × 9 kcal) + (1 × 4 kcal) = 31 kcal

Ratio 2:1
Each dietary unit = 2 g fat and 1 g protein and carbohydrate
Energy content of each dietary unit = (2 × 9 kcal) + (1 × 4 kcal) = 22 kcal

---

Box 8.2   Example calculation of a classical KD prescription using the dietary unit method

Subject
4-year-old girl, ambulant
Weight 16 kg (50th centile)
EAR 1460 kcal
KD calories = 90% × 1460 = 1314 kcal/day
Protein 16 g (1 g/kg body weight)

4:1 ratio KD
40 kcal per dietary unit
Dietary units = 1314/40 = 33 diet units daily
Fat = 33 × 4 = 132 g
Protein and carbohydrate = 33 × 1 = 33 g
Protein = 16 g
Carbohydrate = 33 − 16 = 17 g
Per meal if having four meals a day: 132/4 = 33 g fat; 16/4 = 4 g protein; 17/4 = 4.25 g
  (can round down to 4.2 g) carbohydrate
NB: if using the modified exchange list method (see later in chapter) this can be rational-
  ized to 4 g for ease of calculation)

Thus 33 g fat to 8.2 g protein + carbohydrate = 4:1

To start diet at a 2:1 ratio
Per meal if having four meals a day: fat 33 g; protein 4 g; carbohydrate 4.2 g as food
  (with an extra 8 g of carbohydrate as fruit juice) = 12.2 g
Thus 33 g fat to 16.2 g protein + carbohydrate = 2:1

**To increase the diet ratio to 3:1 (may wish to increase more slowly at
0.5 of a ratio at each ratio change)**
Per meal if having four meals a day: fat 33 g; protein 4 g; carbohydrate 4.2 g as food (with
  an extra 3 g of carbohydrate as fruit juice) = 7.2 g
Thus 33 g fat to 11.2 g protein + carbohydrate = 3:1
Gradually work up the ratios until the necessary ketosis is achieved

A practical way of initiating the diet is to calculate the meals and snacks as a 4:1 diet ratio and temporarily reduce this ratio to 2:1 using carbohydrate in the form of extra fruit juice (will increase calories slightly in the short term). As the ratio increases the food prescription stays the same but the fruit juice is removed as necessary.

Meal planning

Having calculated the amounts of fat, protein and carbohydrate for each meal, this needs to be translated into food. Each meal or snack must be in the same ratio. Recipes will need to be calculated for individual meals and snacks. Fortunately, good computer programs are available such as Electronic Ketogenic Manager (EKM) or Ketoplanner which both dietitians and parents can use. Programs are available free to download for dietitians and for parents (with their dietitian's consent). Further information can be found at www.edm2000.com. Computer programs offer accuracy and allow a wider variety of foods to be incorporated in the diet.

Using the amounts taken from the calculated example for a 4:1 classical KD, meal recipes have been calculated using EKM (Box 8.3). These recipes all aim at a similar prescription, but contain very small differences in carbohydrate and protein content. These are not important when you consider the following.

1 The values in the food tables on which the calculations are based are an average of several samples of each individual food item.
2 The food when cooked will be transformed differently every time it is cooked; even small temperature fluctuations can make a difference.
3 There will always be some residue on cooking utensils, plates and children's hands and faces.

Creating meals from the ingredients allowed requires skill and imagination. Training and guidance must be given on how to use the foods (see examples in Box 8.4). Once families start thinking and understanding the concept of high-fat cookery, they devise many more ideas of their own. Sources of advice and support are essential such as an experienced dietitian and parental websites, for example Matthew's Friends, which also gives many recipe ideas (www.matthewsfriends.org).

After a few weeks or months (if not done before) the meals and menus can be expanded and become more adventurous. The dietitian can supply the necessary recipes for this or families may wish to use the computer program themselves to calculate meals if the dietitian is happy for them to do so. These more complicated meals make computer programs an essential tool for all concerned in making the now-established diet palatable and therefore sustainable. Ultimately the choice of how the diet meals and menus are calculated on behalf of the patients involved is a decision made by their dietitian.

Box 8.3   Example 4:1 ratio recipes for the classical KD, based on figures from calculation in Box 8.2

Scrambled egg and tomato meal (breakfast idea)

Olive oil	11 g
Butter	12 g
Double cream	20 g
Eggs, chicken, raw	25 g
Tomatoes, raw (chopped)	40 g
Strawberries	32 g

- Fry the chopped tomato in the olive oil. Melt the butter in a saucepan and add the double cream and beaten egg.
- Serve the strawberries sliced separately.

Using EKM, this provides 332 kcal, 33.4 g fat, 4 g protein, 3.8 g carbohydrate.

Steak meal

Raw rump beef steak	12 g
Butter	19 g
Raw tomatoes	45 g
Double cream	33 g
Raspberries	40 g

- Cook steak in butter, serve with tomatoes. Serve raspberries and cream for dessert.

Using EKM, this provides 329 kcal, 33 g fat, 4 g protein, 4.2 g carbohydrate.

Frankfurter and mash

Swede, boiled	45 g
Carrots, boiled	35 g
Butter	18 g
Double cream	25 g
Frankfurter sausage	25 g

- Mash the swede and carrot with butter and some of the double cream and serve with the Frankfurter sausage.
- The remaining double cream can be served with sugar-free jelly.

Using EKM, this provides 332 kcal, 33 g fat, 4.3 g protein, 3.8 g carbohydrate.

Ratatouille

Olive oil	19 g
Onion, raw	5 g
Green pepper, raw	20 g
Tomatoes, canned	30 g
Courgette, raw	30 g
Aubergine, raw	51 g
Parmesan cheese, fresh	6 g
Double cream	25 g

- Heat the oil in a saucepan, add the vegetables and soften.
- Place the vegetables in a small dish and add the Parmesan cheese, cook in a medium oven for about 20 minutes.
- Serve the double cream with a sugar-free jelly.

Using EKM, this provides 332 kcal, 33.2 g fat, 4.1 g protein, 4.2 g carbohydrate.

Cauliflower and broccoli cheese

Double cream	18 g
Cheddar cheese, grated	8 g
Broccoli, cooked in water	25 g
Cauliflower, cooked in water	25 g
Olive oil	21 g
Strawberries	45 g

- Mix double cream and olive oil with the grated cheese, heat gently in a small saucepan until the cheese melts.
- Pour the sauce over the cooked broccoli and cauliflower.
- Serve the strawberries alone or with sugar-free jelly.

Using EKM, this provides 329 kcal, 32.9 g fat, 4.2 g protein, 4 g carbohydrate.

Cod in mushroom and cream sauce

Cod, raw	10 g
Olive oil	18 g
Broccoli cooked	25 g
Mushrooms, raw	30 g
Double cream	30 g
Raspberries	56 g

- Fry the cod in olive oil for a few minutes, add the mushrooms and cook until tender. Add double cream and heat through.
- The broccoli can be added or served separately.
- Serve sugar-free jelly with raspberries.

Using EKM, this provides 329 kcal, 33 g fat, 4.3 g protein, 3.8 g carbohydrate.

Box 8.4   Practical advice on how to use double cream and butter

Double cream
- Whip and flavour with carbohydrate-free vanilla essence and freeze = ice cream.
- Whip into sugar-free jelly = mousse.
- Liquidize with fruit, e.g. raspberries and water = smoothie or freeze as an ice lolly.
- Whip into a whirl on top of sugar-free jelly containing chopped fruit = trifle.
- Mix with herbs or spices, warm and pour over meat, chicken or fish.

Butter
- Melt over vegetables.
- Flavour with herbs or garlic and use to cook meat or fish.
- Mix with grated cheese and use as topping for meat or fish which can be baked or grilled.

Ketoshake meal replacements

If a child is unwell and needs a meal replacement, the aim is to replace a meal with a similar prescription made up in a drink, which may be more acceptable when ill. Ideally the use of a complete ketogenic product such as those available for enteral feeds (see Chapter 14) would be an easy option. However, this type pf product has a fixed ketogenic ratio, usually 4:1, and may not therefore be suitable for children whose diets are a different ratio. Alternatives can be made from double cream or Calogen (Nutricia) mixed with a protein source, such as Protifar (Nutricia) or Vitapro (Vitaflo), and a carbohydrate source, such as fresh fruit or Maxijul (Nutricia). This can be mixed together, or liquidized if fruit is used, and water added to individual tolerance or taste. This mixture does not have added electrolytes or vitamins and minerals and is therefore not suitable for long-term use. It is a meal replacement to be used for no more than 24 hours. An example recipe is given in Table 8.3, aiming to produce a 4:1 ratio drink which has the same prescription as the recipe examples in Box 8.3.

An alternative method for implementing a classical KD that uses exchanges

Meal planning may be done using exchange lists for fat, protein and carbohydrate. These are not standardized but individual to each centre. Tables 8.4, 8.5 and 8.6 give examples of exchanges for protein, fat and carbohydrate. Values for these exchanges were calculated from *McCance and Widdowson's The Composition of Foods*, 6th edition (Food Standards Agency, 2002).

Table 8.3   Example recipe for a classical KD meal replacement drink (figures in parentheses refer to amounts if using Vitapro as a protein source rather than Protifar).

Product	Protein (g)	Fat (g)	Carbohydrate (g)
3 g Protifar (or 4 g Vitapro)	2.7	0	0
	(3)	(trace)	(0.4)
2.5 g Maxijul (or reduce to 2 g if	0	0	2.4
using Vitapro as protein source)	(0)	(0)	(1.9)
68 g double cream*	1.2	33	1.8
Totals†	3.9	33	4.2
	(4.2)	(33)	(4.1)

*Double cream values are those provided on the product label as food table values are not accurate for most UK double cream varieties.
†Add water to taste approximately 200 mL.

Table 8.4 Selected protein exchanges for classical KD (average 3 g protein per exchange).

Raw red meat*	15 g
Cooked red meat*	10 g
Raw bacon	20 g
Cooked bacon	15 g
Raw white fish	15 g
Cooked white fish	15 g
Raw turkey	15 g
Cooked turkey	10 g
Raw chicken	15 g
Cooked chicken	10 g
Raw egg	½ egg
Cheddar type cheese†	12 g
Tuna fish or salmon tinned in oil	12 g

*Red meat does not include offal; in particular liver is to be avoided as it contains too much vitamin A to be safe on a KD.
†The average fat per protein exchange is less than 1.0 g without including cheese and egg which contain 3–4 g of fat per exchange, but it is not usually necessary to count this.
Average carbohydrate content is negligible.

Table 8.5 Selected fat exchanges for classical KD (average 15 g fat per exchange).

Butter	20 g
Margarine (containing 75% fat)	20 g
Oil	15 g
Mayonnaise*	20 g
Calogen	30 mL
Double cream (not Elmlea)†*	30 g

*The average carbohydrate content per exchange is 0.2 g, except for double cream and mayonnaise. Mayonnaise contains 0.3 g carbohydrate per 20 g dependent on the brand used. Double cream contains 0.8 g of carbohydrate per 30 g depending on the brand used. The values for double cream are taken from product information. The value in *McCance and Widdowson's The Composition of Foods*, 6th edition, although an average of double cream, includes Jersey cream which is much higher in fat and therefore the average fat is too high for our calculations. Most households will use a supermarket double cream not Jersey cream.
†The average protein per exchange is negligible, except for the protein content of double cream, which is approximately 0.5 g of protein per 30 g depending on the brand used.

Training and guidance must be given on how to use the foods listed in the exchanges. Although this method will not be as accurate as calculating recipes from food tables, it is considerably less time-consuming for both the dietitian and family. The other benefit is that the exchange system can be taught to the family, giving them a real understanding of how the diet calculations work. This means that when ratio changes are made they can implement these themselves. They are also able to

Table 8.6   Selected carbohydrate exchanges for classical KD (average 2 g carbohydrate per exchange).

Fruit*	
Apple	20 g
Banana	8 g
Blackberries	40 g
Blackcurrants	30 g
Grapes	13 g
Grapefruit	30 g
Gooseberries (stewed without sugar)	80 g
Kiwi fruit	18 g
Mango	14 g
Melon	36 g
Orange	24 g
Orange juice	18 g
Peach	26 g
Pear	20 g
Raspberries	44 g
Strawberries	34 g
Vegetables[†]	
Beetroot cooked (pickled)	36 g
Cabbage cooked	90 g
Carrots cooked	46 g
Carrots raw	34 g
Cauliflower cooked	96 g
Leeks boiled	76 g
Peas, frozen, boiled	20 g
Tomato raw	64 g
Turnip cooked	100 g

*The average protein content of each fruit exchange is 0.2 g; fat content is negligible.
[†]Each vegetable exchange contains an average of 0.9 g protein and 0.3 g fat.

have a wider choice of menus as they do not have to ask the dietitian to calculate every menu change. The exchange system may be particularly useful when the KD is commenced, as a means to try a more flexible approach initially and give a family independence to vary the diet simply using the exchange lists to suit their own preferences. If exchanges are a success and the KD is effective in controlling seizures, then after the usual 3-month trial the family or caregivers should be offered training on using a recognized computer program to calculate meals and recipes.

Our experience of using exchanges is that for most patients they are restrictive enough to give an effective ketosis; where this is not the case then more dietetic input is needed and a computer program can be used to restrict the diet further. Families using a computer program after using the exchange system will have a basic grounding in nutrition and know which foods contain fat, protein and carbohydrate; they will then be better able to use the programs. Although there will be differences in the amounts of foods allowed when comparing KD meals that have been planned by the exchange system method and the recipe calculation method, this type of difference does not seem to affect the level of ketosis, not surprising in the light of the reported success of the more flexible modified Atkins diet which only measures carbohydrate and does not measure fat or protein (see Chapter 10). Both methods can be used to adjust the diet as and when fine tuning is needed (see Chapter 17).

Conclusion

Although classical KD prescriptions are calculated using principles developed nearly 80 years ago, the development of computer programs and exchange lists have greatly reduced the time taken to turn these prescriptions into recipes and meal plans, allowing more flexibility and inclusion of a wider variety of foods. Whether the stricter regimen of the classical KD has efficacy benefits over the more liberal modified diets is subject to ongoing debate (Kossoff et al., 2010), but it is still the most appropriate choice of diet therapy for many children with intractable seizures and continues to have an important place as part of the now broader palate of dietary treatments on offer.

References

Department of Health (1991) *Dietary Reference Values for Food Energy and Nutrients for the United Kingdom*. London: HMSO.

Food Standards Agency (2002) *McCance and Widdowson's The Composition of Foods*, 6th summary edn. Cambridge: Royal Society of Chemistry.

Freeman, J.M., Kossoff, E.H., Freeman, J.B. and Kelly, M.T. (2007) *The Ketogenic Diet: A Treatment for Children and Others With Epilepsy*, 4th edn. New York: Demos Medical Publishing.

Kossoff, E.H., Dorward, J.L., Miranda, M.J., Wiemer-Kruel, A., Kang, H.C. and Kim, H.D. (2010) Will seizure control improve by switching from the modified Atkins diet to the traditional ketogenic diet? *Epilepsia* **51**, 2496–2499.

Kossoff, E.H., Freeman, J.M., Turner, Z. and Rubenstein, J.E. (2011) *Ketogenic Diets: Treatments for Epilepsy and Other Disorders*, 5th edn. New York: Demos Medical Publishing.

Neal, E.G. and Magrath, G. (2007) The ketogenic diet. In: Shaw, V. and Lawson, M. (eds) *Clinical Paediatric Dietetics*, 3rd edn. Oxford: Blackwell Publishing Ltd.

Talbot, F.B. (1930) *Treatment of Epilepsy*. New York: Macmillian.

Talbot, F.B., Metcalf, K.M. and Moriarty, M.E. (1927) A clinical study of epileptic children treated by the ketogenic diet. *Boston Medical and Surgical Journal* **196**, 89–96.

World Health Organization (2007) *Protein and Amino Acid Requirements in Human Nutrition: Report of a Joint WHO/FAO/UNU Expert Consultation*. WHO Technical Report Series 935.

Chapter 9

The medium-chain triglyceride ketogenic diet

Elizabeth Neal

Matthew's Friends Charity and Clinics, Lingfield, UK

The medium-chain triglyceride (MCT) ketogenic diet (KD) was first described in the 1970s (Huttenlocher et al., 1971) as a modification of the classical KD; the increased ketogenic potential of MCT allows inclusion of more dietary protein and carbohydrate with the aim of improving palatability and compliance. This chapter explains the calculation of the MCT KD, and the use of exchange lists and recipes to develop a daily meal plan.

Energy prescription

The principles for assessing energy requirements in a child starting the MCT KD are the same as those for the classical KD, and have been covered in the first section of Chapter 8. There is no literature evidence for allowing more dietary energy on the MCT KD; indeed a review of the earlier KD literature for information on the types of prescription used in MCT diets suggests conflicting reports regarding energy prescriptions (Table 9.1). The first paper to compare the two types of KD (Huttenlocher, 1976) did not distinguish between the classical or MCT protocol in terms of total daily dietary energy prescription.

Dietary prescription

- *MCT*. The traditional MCT KD provides 60% of total calories from MCT; an alternative modified (John Radcliffe) version provides 30% of energy from MCT. Both protocols have limitations: the former can cause gastrointestinal tolerance problems, the latter a poor ketosis. In practice, a starting level of

Dietary Treatment of Epilepsy: Practical Implementation of Ketogenic Therapy,
First Edition. Edited by Elizabeth Neal.
© 2012 John Wiley & Sons, Ltd. Published 2012 by John Wiley & Sons, Ltd.

Table 9.1 Summary of studies reporting MCT KD treatment.

Reference	Number in study	Age range	Energy prescription	Diet prescription*	Translating into meals
Berman (1978)	18	2–17 years	60–75 kcal/kg	19% CHO, 10% protein, 11% LCT, 60% MCT	Not stated
Clark and House (1978)	13	Not stated	Recommended daily allowance (UK)	60% MCT, 40% from other food sources	100 kcal and 50 kcal exchanges
Huttenlocher et al. (1971)	12	2.5–16 years	Recommended daily allowance (USA)	19% CHO, 10% protein, 11% LCT, aiming for 60% MCT	Protein, carbohydrate and fat exchanges
Huttenlocher (1976)	18	18 months to 18 years	'Low maintenance' (75 kcal/kg), increased as needed	18% CHO, 10% protein, 12% LCT, 60% MCT	Not stated
Mak et al. (1999)	13	3–13 years	110% of recommended daily requirement (Tawain)	1.5–2 g protein/kg daily, <19% CHO, 65–70% MCT, not less than 10% LCT	Not stated
Ross et al. (1985)	9	3 months to 13 years	'Recommended total calories for age' (USA)	'Protein 1–1.5 g/kg, remaining energy in 3:1 ratio of fat: CHO, with 60% of total energy as MCT'= ~5–8% protein, 12% CHO and 80% fat (60% MCT; 20% LCT)	Not stated
Schwartz et al. (1989)	55 children and 4 adults	20 under 5 years 25 aged 5–10 years 9 aged 11–15 years 5 aged 15–54 years	Recommended daily allowance (UK)	19% CHO, 10% protein, 11% LCT, 60% MCT Modified diet (N=13): 19% CHO, 10% protein, 30% MCT, 41% LCT	Protein and carbohydrate exchanges
Sills et al. (1986)	50	2–15 years	'Assessed on individual basis by dietitian'	Aiming for 60% MCT	Not stated
Trauner (1985)	17	12 months to 13 years	'Total calorie needs calculated': energy intake gradually increased to ~150% of needs to prevent weight loss	60% MCT, 15% protein, 15% CHO, 10% LCT	Not stated

*%, percentage of total dietary energy from macronutrient; CHO, carbohydrate; LCT, long-chain triglyceride from food sources; MCT, medium-chain triglyceride.

40–55 % energy from MCT provides a good balance between tolerance and adequate ketosis. The ideal percentage can depend on age (younger child may need less to establish a good ketosis), tolerance and current dietary preferences. The MCT can be increased or decreased as needed during fine-tuning (see Chapter 17). The energy content per gram of MCT itself is an unresolved issue. Current European Union guidelines state that the standard conversion factor for fat of 9 kcal/g should be used and in the UK most MCT products are labelled accordingly. Literature reports suggest that studies on the MCT diet have used the widely accepted lower value of 8.3 kcal/g. Other work suggests an even lower value of 7 kcal/g may be more accurate (Ranhotra et al., 1995). For the example calculations used in this chapter the value of 8.3 kcal/g has been chosen.

- *Carbohydrate*. This usually provides 15–18 % of total dietary energy.
- *Protein*. This provides 10 % of total dietary energy (up to 12 % may be needed in older non-ambulant children with very low energy requirements, in order to meet estimated protein requirements).
- *Long-chain triglyceride (LCT)*. This provides the remaining dietary energy (about 20–30 % of total, depending on the percentage of energy from MCT, protein and carbohydrate).

This division of energy in the MCT KD provides a ketogenic ratio of approximately 1.2 : 1 to 1.6 : 1 (depending on amount of protein and carbohydrate prescribed).

Daily meal plan

The dietary prescription must be translated into meals (and snacks if required) that will suit the individual child. The following steps should be worked through.

1 Discuss the ideal daily number of meals and snacks so that the prescription can be tailored to an individual preference.
2 Divide up the total prescribed daily MCT between meals and snacks. This can be provided by MCT oil or the emulsion Liquigen (50 % MCT/50 % water) (both Nutricia); these are available on prescription in the UK. Liquigen can either be used in recipes or added to milk (could be skimmed or semi-skimmed depending on the amount of LCT needed in the diet). A bedtime drink or snack containing MCT will help maintain ketosis overnight. Acceptance of a milk/MCT mixture frequently decreases with time on the diet. Other ways to use MCT are to incorporate Liquigen into a sugar-free jelly, add to soup, mix into mashed potato, use to make a sauce or in other recipes. MCT oil can also be used in a range of recipes, but note that MCT has a lower flashpoint than LCT so care must be taken when frying with MCT oil, keeping the temperature fairly low.
3 Determine a total milk allowance for the day, again based on individual dietary preferences such as how much milk a child currently drinks or uses on cereal.

4 Subtract the amount of carbohydrate that will be provided by the milk allowance from the total daily carbohydrate allowance; the rest can be given as carbohydrate exchanges (Table 9.2). These exchanges must be divided up evenly over the day, and none should be given without a source of MCT at the same meal or snack. Because there is wide variation in carbohydrate content between different foods (e.g. it is much lower in vegetables than in pasta and rice), exchanges are listed that provide either 10, 5 or 1 g carbohydrate. These can be used in different combinations providing the total amount of carbohydrate is equal to that prescribed for a particular meal or snack.

5 Subtract the amount of protein that will be provided by the milk allowance from the total daily protein allowance. The remaining can be given as high biological value fat-adjusted protein exchanges (Box 9.1). These should also be divided up over the day (although this is not as important as it is for the carbohydrate exchanges). Although some protein will be additionally provided by the carbohydrate exchanges, this is generally of low biological value and usually amounts to no more than 5–10 g daily. This amount is not included in the protein calculation, but may need to be considered during dietary fine tuning if a reduction in protein is necessary.

6 Subtract the amount of LCT that will be provided by the milk allowance from the total daily LCT allowance, then also subtract the amount of fat that will be provided by the fat-adjusted high biological value protein exchanges. This is averaged at 3 g fat per exchange (see additional considerations below). The remaining amount of LCT can be given as fat exchanges (Box 9.2). Again these should also be divided up over the day if possible.

7 Full vitamin/mineral/trace element supplementation should be given. Check the amount of milk, cheese and other dairy products in the diet to determine whether additional calcium supplementation is needed.

8 Prescribing an exact amount of MCT and number of each type of exchange for each meal or snack makes them easier to use and allows a more accurate daily balance of MCT and macronutrients (see worked example in Box 9.3). Recipes can then be devised using these exchanges (see ideas in Box 9.4). Exact recipes can be used on the MCT diet and families who are familiar with Electronic Ketogenic Manager (EKM) or other computer programs may prefer to use them. Snacks can be suggested using half exchanges, but it is often easier to give snacks as calculated recipes, containing a prescribed amount of MCT (see examples in Box 9.5). Further recipe ideas can be found at www.matthewsfriends.org.

Additional considerations relating to use of exchange lists

- Prescribed values of carbohydrate, protein and fat will often need to be rounded up or down to the nearest half number of exchanges to allow for ease of use (as in Box 9.3).

Table 9.2   Example of selected carbohydrate exchanges for MCT ketogenic diet.

	1 g carbohydrate exchange	5 g carbohydrate exchange	10 g carbohydrate exchange
Vegetables (g)			
Broccoli, raw	56	278	
Broccoli, boiled	91	455	
Cabbage, boiled, average	45	227	
Carrots, raw	17	83	
Carrots, boiled	23	114	
Cauliflower, boiled	48	238	
Celeriac, raw	43	217	
Celery, raw	111	556	
Courgette, raw	56	278	
Cucumber	57	285	
French beans, boiled	34	172	
Leeks, boiled	38	192	
Lettuce, average, raw	59	294	
Mushrooms, common, raw	250		
Onions, raw	13	63	
Onions, spring	33	167	
Peas, frozen, boiled	10	52	
Peppers, green, raw	38	192	
Peppers, red, raw	16	78	
Runner beans, boiled	43	217	
Sweetcorn kernels, boiled	5	26	
Tomato purée	7	35	
Tomatoes, raw	32	161	
Potatoes, old boiled		29	59
Rice, pasta, cereals, bread and biscuits (g)			
Rice, white, easy cook, boiled		16	32
Rice brown, boiled		16	31
Spaghetti, white, boiled		23	45
Spaghetti, wholemeal, boiled		22	43
Cornflakes		6	12
Rice Krispies		6	11
Weetabix		7	13
Bread, white, sliced		11	22
Bread, wholemeal, average		12	24
Digestive biscuits, plain		7	15
Fruits (g)			
Apples, cooking, stewed no sugar	12	62	123
Apples, eating	8	42	85
Banana	4	22	43
Blackberries	20	98	196
Blackcurrants	15	76	152
Cherries	11	53	105
Kiwi fruit	9	47	94
Oranges	12	59	118
Peaches	13	66	132
Pears	10	50	100
Plums, raw, average	11	57	114
Raspberries	22	109	217
Rhubarb, stewed no sugar	143	714	1429
Strawberries	17	83	167

Box 9.1   Example of protein exchanges for MCT ketogenic diet (fat-adjusted).
Each of the following provides 6 g of protein and an average 3 g of fat.

Fish
White fish (e.g. cod, coley, plaice, haddock, whiting): 30 g, with an extra 3 g oil or 4 g
    butter, margarine or mayonnaise (weighed raw, baked, poached, grilled or steamed)
Herring, kipper or mackerel: 30 g (weighed raw, grilled or smoked)
Salmon: 30 g (weighed raw or steamed)
Smoked salmon: 24 g, with an extra 2 g oil or 3 g butter, margarine or mayonnaise
Salmon, pink, canned: 25 g
Pilchards or sardines, canned in tomato sauce: 35 g
Sardines, canned in oil or brine: 28 g
Tuna, canned in oil: 22 g

Meat
Bacon: 38 g if weighed raw or 25 g if weighed grilled or fried
Ham: 33 g, with an extra 2 g oil or 3 g butter, margarine or mayonnaise
Gammon: 26 g (weighed boiled)
Beef: 28 g if weighed raw or 20 g if weighed cooked (grilled, stewed, fried, roasted or
    barbecued)
Corned beef, canned: 23 g
Lamb: 30 g if weighed raw or 23 g grilled chops or 21 g roast lamb or 25 g stewed lamb
Pork: 32 g if weighed raw or 20 g if weighed cooked (grilled, stewed, fried, roasted or
    barbecued)
Mince (beef or lamb): 30 g (weighed raw or cooked)
Chicken: 27 g if weighed raw, with an extra 3 g oil or 4 g butter, margarine or mayonnaise.
    Cooked chicken breast: 20 g, with an extra 2 g oil or 3 g butter, margarine or
    mayonnaise. Cooked chicken leg: 25 g
Turkey: 27 g if weighed raw, with an extra 3 g oil or 4 g butter, margarine or mayonnaise.
    Cooked turkey breast: 18 g, with an extra 3 g oil or 4 g butter, margarine or mayonnaise.
    Cooked turkey leg: 21 g, with an extra 2 g oil or 3 g butter, margarine or mayonnaise
Salami: 29 g

Cheese
Cheddar: 24 g
Cottage (not low fat): 47 g
Edam: 23 g
Brie: 30 g
Stilton: 25 g
Parmesan: 17 g

Other
Eggs: 1 medium (~50 g if weighed boiled or poached)
Quorn: 45 g

- All food should be weighed.
- Foods that contain both carbohydrate and protein will often need to be included, for example yoghurt, fromage frais, fish fingers, fish cakes, baked beans and sausages. Using food product values, exchanges for these foods can be worked out, but because of the differences in composition between different brands of a product, it is best that this is calculated on an individual basis depending on the brand used.

Box 9.2   Example of fat exchanges for MCT ketogenic diet. Each of the following provides 5 g of fat.

6g butter: any type, e.g. Anchor, Country Life, supermarkets own brand (not lighter versions)

5g oil: a vegetable oil, such as olive or sunflower, is recommended

6g mayonnaise: Hellmans (jar) or alternative full fat

8g margarine: not low-fat spreads

10g double cream: not UHT spray creams or imitation creams like Elmlea which are lower in fat

20g full fat Philadelphia cream cheese

10g Mascarpone cheese

The following foods can be used as fat exchanges, but will contribute carbohydrate and/ or protein to the diet so include a maximum of one or two of these 5-g fat exchanges daily

25g avocado pear

7g walnuts, coconut, pecan nuts, pine nuts or brazil nuts

8g hazelnuts

9g almonds or pistachio nuts (roasted and salted)

11g plain peanuts

8g roasted and salted peanuts

8g sesame seeds

6g macadamia nuts

- Protein exchanges are averaged at 3 g fat per 6 g protein exchange; however, extra fat in the form of oil or butter is only added to the exchange if the fat content is 1.2 g or under per exchange. Some exchanges, for example cheese and oily fish, have a much higher fat content which is not accounted for in the diet. If the protein sources in an individual diet are primarily from high-fat foods, an adjustment to the number of additional fat exchanges needed could be made to reduce dietary energy.
- All the listed exchanges are based on *McCance and Widdowson's The Composition of Foods*, 6th edition (Food Standards Agency, 2002). It is recommended that individual food product labels are checked to ensure they are consistent with these values for carbohydrate, protein and fat.
- Although some centres prefer to use calorie exchanges, the use of separate carbohydrate, protein and fat exchanges is recommended as this gives a more even macronutrient distribution over the meals and snacks.

Introduction of the MCT

On commencing the MCT KD, the MCT dose needs to be built up slowly (over about 5–10 days), as it may cause abdominal discomfort, vomiting or diarrhoea if introduced rapidly. During this introduction period the rest of the diet can be given as prescribed, but an extra meal may be needed to make up the calories while using less MCT.

Box 9.3   Example calculation of an MCT KD

Subject
Boy, 3 years old, weight 14.5 kg (approximately 50th centile)
Estimated average requirement (EAR) 1380 kcal
Diet history approximately 1220 kcal daily
Energy prescription = 1300 kcal (average of diet history and EAR)

Calculation of dietary prescription
45% energy from MCT = 585 kcal = 70.5 g MCT oil or 141 g Liquigen (round down to 70 g
    MCT oil or 140 g Liquigen)
15% energy from carbohydrate = 195 kcal = 48.8 g
10% energy from protein = 130 kcal = 32.5 g
Remaining 30% energy from fat in foods = 390 kcal = 43.3 g

Translating the prescription into a daily plan
1 Milk allowance = 300 mL semi-skimmed milk = 14.1 g carbohydrate, 10.2 g protein,
   5.1 g fat
2 Carbohydrate (aiming for 48.8 g daily): subtract 14.1 g (milk allowance) = 34.7 g. This
   can be rounded up to 35 g
3 Protein (aiming for 32.5 g daily): subtract 10.2 g (milk allowance) = 22.3 g. This can be
   rounded down to 21 g = 3.5 × 6 g exchanges
4 Fat (aiming for 43.3 g daily): subtract 5.1 g (milk allowance) and subtract 10.5 g
   (3.5 × 3 g from fat-adjusted protein exchanges) = 27.7 g. This can be rounded down to
   27.5 g = 5.5 × 5 g fat exchanges

Summary daily plan
70 g MCT oil *or* 140 g Liquigen
300 mL semi-skimmed milk
35 g carbohydrate (divided up over the day using 10 g, 5 g or 1 g exchanges)
3.5 × 6 g fat-adjusted protein exchanges
5.5 × 5 g fat exchanges

Suggested structure over the day
• *Breakfast*: 20 g MCT oil *or* 40 g Liquigen, 150 mL semi-skimmed milk, 10 g carbohy-
  drate, 6 g protein (1 exchange), 5 g LCT (1 fat exchange)
• *Lunch and tea*: 18 g MCT oil *or* 36 g Liquigen, 10 g carbohydrate, 6 g protein
  (1 exchange), 10 g LCT (2 fat exchanges)
• *Snack* (could be used mid-morning or afternoon): 5 g MCT oil *or* 10 g Liquigen, 5 g
  carbohydrate, 3 g protein (1/2 protein exchange) and 2.5 g LCT (1/2 fat exchange)
• *Before bed drink*: 150 mL semi-skimmed milk (as a milk drink) mixed with 18 g Liquigen

Ketoshake meal replacements

Just as with the classical KD, if a child is unwell and unable to eat the ketogenic
food, a meal replacement 'ketoshake' may be more acceptable. This drink can be
made up to the normal meal prescription using a blended mix of Liquigen, milk,
double cream and fruit. This can be sipped throughout the day as needed, but as

---

Box 9.4   Example MCT KD menu (based on daily structure in Box 9.3)

Scrambled egg breakfast
24 g wholemeal bread (10 g carbohydrate exchange), toasted
1 egg (1 protein exchange); whisk with 40 g Liquigen and 6 g butter (1 fat exchange)
150 mL semi-skimmed milk drink

Salmon in cheese sauce lunch
20 g salmon (raw weight) (2/3 protein exchange) and 29 g sliced boiled potato (5 g carbohydrate exchange); fry together in 9 g MCT oil with garlic and parsley seasoning.
Sauce: 20 g double cream (2 fat exchanges) mixed with 9 g MCT oil and 8 g cheddar cheese (1/3 protein exchange). Microwave briefly and pour over the salmon.
Serve with 34 g boiled French beans (1 g carbohydrate exchange) and 23 g boiled carrot (1 g carbohydrate exchange).
30 g pear for dessert (3 × 1 g carbohydrate exchanges)

Chicken and vegetable korma tea
27 g raw chicken (1 protein exchange) and 33 g spring onion (1 g carbohydrate exchange); fry both in a mix of 13 g MCT oil and 3 g olive oil (added with chicken protein exchange to fat adjust) with added garlic, mild chilli powder and turmeric spices.
Add 46 g carrot (2 × 1 g carbohydrate exchange), 48 g cauliflower (1 g carbohydrate exchange) and 91 g broccoli (1 g carbohydrate exchange) (all weighed boiled or steamed) to the chicken mix, cook through and add a pinch of chicken Oxo cube, a drop of sweetener and lemon or lime juice.
Slowly stir in 9 g ground almonds (1 fat exchange) and 10 g double cream (1 fat exchange), and 10 g Liquigen, adding extra water as required.
42 g apple for dessert (5 g carbohydrate exchange)

---

there are no added vitamins, minerals or trace elements it should not be used as a complete food source for more than 24 hours.

Conclusion

The MCT KD allows a generous carbohydrate prescription and can therefore be a useful alternative to the classical KD and modified Atkins diet with their stricter carbohydrate restrictions. Introducing the MCT gradually and then making regular adjustments as part of the fine-tuning process will ensure optimal balance between tolerance and dietary efficacy.

Acknowledgements

Val Aldridge at Matthews Friends for her ideas and advice on the recipes; Sue Wood for her carbohydrate exchanges.

Box 9.5   Example snack recipes (each of the following provides 5 g MCT, 5 g carbohydrate, 3 g protein and 2.5 g fat, based on daily structure in Box 9.3)

Cake/biscuit snack ideas
These cake/biscuit recipes can be made in batches by multiplying up the ingredients and making a large batch at once. They can then be divided up into individual portions and frozen for use as needed. To sweeten, use Hermesetas liquid or Sweetex or saccharin tablets dissolved in a drop of water. To sweeten a batch of 10 recipes you will probably need about five tablets or a few drops of Hermesetas liquid.

Raspberry and bran biscuits
7 g raspberries
9 g All Bran
4 g ground almonds
8 g egg white
5 g MCT oil
Sweetener
Mix all ingredients and bake for 20 minutes (gas mark 5–6)

Chocolate cake
7 g wholemeal flour
13 g egg
2 g cocoa powder
1 g desiccated coconut
5 g MCT oil or 10 g Liquigen
Sweetener
Mix all ingredients and bake for 15 minutes (gas mark 5–6)

Other snack ideas
Bananas and bacon
21 g banana
15 g back bacon raw (fat trimmed)
3 g double cream
5 g MCT oil
Wrap bacon over banana, pour oil over and bake low and slow. Add cream to serve.

Fruit meringue
21 g egg white
4 g desiccated coconut
30 g raspberries
30 g strawberries
20 g blueberries
5 g MCT oil
Sweetener
Whisk egg white until stiff, mix all ingredients together (enough to fill two muffin cups) and bake for 15 minutes (gas mark 5–6).

Fruit milkshake
80 g semi-skimmed milk
2 g double cream
10 g Liquigen
25 g raspberries *or* 20 g strawberries
Purée/blend fruit, mix all ingredients, serve chilled.

Egg custard
20 g egg (raw weight)
10 g Liquigen
100 g raspberries *or* 80 g strawberries *or* 40 g apple *or* 20 g banana
Mix Liquigen and egg and cook in microwave or oven (approximately 25 minutes, medium heat) until set. Serve with fruit.

Fruit ice cream
25 g raspberries *or* 20 g strawberries
3 g double cream
80 g semi-skimmed milk
10 g Liquigen
Mix all ingredients together and freeze, stir after 1 hour.

References

Berman, W. (1978) Medium chain triglycerides in the treatment of intractable childhood epilepsy. *Dev Med Child Neurol* **20**, 249–250.

Clark, B.J. and House, F.M. (1978) Medium chain triglyceride oil ketogenic diets in the treatment of childhood epilepsy. *J Hum Nutr* **32**, 111–116.

Food Standards Agency (2002) *McCance and Widdowson's The Composition of Foods*, 6th summary edn. Cambridge: Royal Society of Chemistry.

Huttenlocher, P.R. (1976) Ketonaemia and seizures: metabolic and anticonvulsant effects of two ketogenic diets in childhood epilepsy. *Pediatr Res* **10**, 536–540.

Huttenlocher, P.R., Wilbourne, A.J. and Sigmore, J.M. (1971) Medium chain triglycerides as a therapy for intractable childhood epilepsy. *Neurology* **21**, 1097–1103.

Mak, S.C., Chi, C.S. and Wan, C.J. (1999) Clinical experience of ketogenic diet on children with refractory epilepsy. *Acta Paediatr Taiwan* **40**, 97–100.

Ranhotra, G.S., Gelroth, J.A. and Glaser, B.K. (1995) Levels of medium-chain triglycerides and their energy value. *Cereal Chem* **72**, 365–367.

Ross, D.L., Swainman, K.F., Torres, F. and Hansen, J. (1985) Early biochemical and EEG correlates of the ketogenic diet in children with atypical absence epilepsy. *Pediatr Neurol* **1**, 104–108.

Schwartz, R.H., Eaton, J., Bower, B.D. and Aynsley-Green, A. (1989) Ketogenic diets in the tretment of epilepsy: short term clinical effects. *Dev Med Child Neurol* **31**, 145–151.

Sills, M.A., Forsythe, W.I., Haidukewych, D., MacDonald, A. and Robinson, M. (1986) The medium chain triglyceride diet and intractable epilepsy. *Arch Dis Child* **61**, 1168–1172.

Trauner, D.A. (1985) Medium chain triglyceride diet in intractable seizure disorders. *Neurology* **35**, 237–238.

Chapter 10

The modified Atkins diet

Gwyneth Magrath[1], Mary-Anne Leung[2]
and Tara Randall[2]

[1]*Matthew's Friends Charity and Clinics, Lingfield, UK*
[2]*Evelina Children's Hospital, London, UK*

The modified Atkins diet (MAD) has been used by Eric Kossoff and his team at Johns Hopkins Hospital since 2003 (Kossoff et al., 2003); his group were the first to report its success as an alternative to the traditional ketogenic diet (KD) in treating children with epilepsy (Kossoff et al., 2006). Like all the diets used for the treatment of intractable epileptic seizures it is high in fat and restricted in carbohydrate. The great advantage of this regimen is that it is easier to implement and comply with than either the classical KD or the medium-chain triglyceride (MCT) KD. Constipation, weight loss and acidosis are also said to be less of a problem (Kossoff et al., 2011a). This chapter describes how the MAD is implemented, firstly using the Johns Hopkins protocol and then using an alternative approach based on food choices.

The Johns Hopkins MAD protocol

Diet prescription

Protein

Protein is allowed freely. It is neither weighed nor measured and does not necessarily have to be eaten at each meal. It is worth noting that because protein foods are generally considered to be more palatable than those high in fat, advice should be given to ensure that they are not eaten to excess, or the ensuing increase in energy intake could compromise ketosis.

Fat

Foods high in fat are actively encouraged and must be eaten with each meal. The amount of fat is not prescribed but sufficient must be eaten to achieve the necessary ketosis for seizure control. Increasing fat intake may improve efficacy: Kossoff and his team found that using 300 mL daily of a 20% solution of the 4 : 1 ratio ketogenic formula feed Ketocal (Nutricia) in the first month of treatment improved the efficacy of the MAD from 50 to 80% (Kossoff et al., 2011b). A drink of 300 mL Ketocal was given daily which increased dietary fat intake by 43.8 g and the diet ratio from 1.1 : 1 to 1.8 : 1. At this stage the carbohydrate in the Ketocal was not counted as part of the daily carbohydrate allowance. Alternatively, this increase in dietary fat intake could be achieved by giving more fat as food or high-fat drinks.

Carbohydrate

Carbohydrate is initially prescribed at 10 g daily for children, 15 g for adolescents if 10 g is too restrictive for them, and 20 g daily for adults. This carbohydrate can be eaten randomly throughout the day. Although any carbohydrate foods can be used, those with a low glycaemic index will be preferable. This carbohydrate allowance only measures the carbohydrate contained in food and it does not include the fibre. All patients and their families are given comprehensive advice on which foods are the most appropriate sources of protein, fat and carbohydrate.

Energy

Dietary energy is not restricted and there is no need for a pre-diet assessment to calculate energy requirements. Although there is no energy prescription, the energy intake is monitored by using weekly weight checks. Weight loss will need to be addressed with an increase in dietary energy and most probably this will require the addition of more fat into the diet. Excessive weight gain may mean a reduction in protein as well as fat.

Vitamins and minerals

A full vitamin and mineral supplement is needed.

Fluid intake

Fluids must be encouraged to help prevent renal stones.

Adjustments after 1 month

1 Carbohydrate: the carbohydrate prescription for a child remains at 10 g daily for 1 month. After the first month the daily allowance is increased by 5 g. Thereafter, further increases to the daily carbohydrate of 5 g are made on a

monthly basis. The final prescribed amount of carbohydrate is dependent on the patient's seizure control. Most children are eventually established on 20 g of carbohydrate daily and adults on 30 g of carbohydrate daily.

2 Fat: Ketocal can now be removed unless the patient enjoys drinking it. This will lower the fat intake and diet ratio, therefore reducing the diet's potential to maintain ketosis. It might be necessary to increase the dietary fat. Protein continues to be allowed freely unless it is being eaten to excess.

3 Introduce low-carbohydrate manufactured products into the diet.

4 Reduce ketone testing: urinary ketone levels should be checked on a daily basis as with a KD (see Chapter 16) for the first month, when they are likely to be high. They then tend to reduce to levels ranging from trace to moderate by 6 months (Kossoff et al., 2011a), with no adverse effect on seizure control. It is recommended that at 6 months ketones only need to be checked weekly.

5 Consider reducing antiepileptic medications: this should be considered if seizure control has improved, in which case less medication may now be needed. Any changes of medication must be made cautiously, with one change at a time. The diet should remain the same whilst such changes are made.

It is important that only one of these changes is made at a time.

Follow-up appointment

A follow-up appointment within the first 3 months of the diet with the neurologist and dietitian should include a full nutritional blood screen and growth check (see Chapter 18) and a dietary review. Using this information the dietitian will make the necessary dietary adjustments required for each patient.

Fine tuning

The amount of carbohydrate in the MAD is already minimal and should not be reduced to improve ketosis. However, an inadequate fat intake can reduce ketosis and should be increased using high-fat foods, Ketocal, or an MCT fat source such as Liquigen or MCT oil (both Nutricia).

The energy intake must be adequate for the patient's age, weight and height and activity level. An excessive intake will reduce ketosis and advice on reducing dietary energy will be necessary. This advice is best given having reviewed the patient's current dietary intake so that such reductions can be made effectively. The ultimate fine-tuning strategy would be to move the patient to the 'higher-dose diet', i.e. the classical KD. In a retrospective cross-centre study this change of diet improved seizure control in 37% of the 27 children who had made this transition (Kossoff et al., 2010).

Further details on the MAD protocol as implemented at the Johns Hopkins Hospital can be found in the fifth edition of *Ketogenic Diets: Treatments for Epilepsy and Other Disorders* (Kossoff et al., 2011a).

Modified Atkins diet in the UK and Ireland

Prior to 2007 dietary therapy used in the UK for the treatment of intractable epilepsy was either the classical KD or the MCT KD (Magrath et al., 2000; Lord and Magrath, 2010). In 2011 dietitians who were members of the Ketogenic Professional Advisory Group of the UK and Ireland (ketoPAG) were asked for information on use of the MAD in their current practice. This was to establish if the MAD or similar regimens were in use in the UK and Ireland. Eight centres responded, of which all but one were prescribing an adapted version of the MAD which they felt was the most appropriate for use within their clinical practice. These adapted versions of the MAD usually include some form of food choice or exchange lists, so appear stricter in terms of implementation than the Johns Hopkins protocol. This has been felt necessary to allow the dietitian to have confidence and control over the diet, especially if ongoing fine tuning is needed or there is limited paediatric neurologist support. The dietitians concerned reported that their patients on this type of MAD became sufficiently ketotic to improve seizure control. The information gathered from theses eight centres is referred to throughout the following text.

Diet prescription (see also worked example and meal plan in Box 10.1 and Box 10.2)

Protein

Protein intake will often be higher than the normal recommended dietary requirements but care must be taken that the amount of protein offered is not excessive. There has been some limited experience of patients over-indulging in protein foods, which has had a negative impact on their ketosis. Initially, recommended protein sources are unprocessed high-protein choices such as chicken, eggs, lamb, beef and fish, avoiding processed foods with added carbohydrates such as fish fingers and sausages. High-protein food choices are made from a list compiled by the dietitian, such as the example in Box 10.3. The majority of the surveyed centres prescribed foods that were high in protein to be eaten at each meal. Two centres advised on the amount of protein to be eaten at each meal using food choice lists and one centre allowed protein to be eaten randomly.

Fat

Fat should be eaten with each meal or snack. The Johns Hopkins MAD protocol advises that high-fat foods eaten at each meal are neither weighed nor measured. All but one of the surveyed centres prescribed the total or the minimum amount of fat to be eaten at each meal using fat choice lists (Box 10.4). This was done to ensure enough fat was eaten to achieve successful ketosis. Only one centre followed the Johns Hopkins protocol, advising which foods high in fat content should be eaten in generous amounts but not weighed at each meal. These foods were taken from lists of foods with a high-fat content such as butter and mayonnaise.

Box 10.1 Worked example of how to calculate a MAD using food choice method.

Subject
Boy, 12 years old
Weight 43.4 kg (75th centile)
Height 155 cm (>75th centile)
Weight: steady

Energy prescription
Estimated average requirement (Department of Health, 1991): 2220 kcal/day
Estimated energy intake (food diary): 1900 kcal/day
Energy prescription: 2000 kcal/day

Protein prescription
Estimated average requirement (Department of Health, 1991): 42 g/day + 30 g to allow for extra eaten
Protein prescription: 72 g/day (288 kcal)

Carbohydrate prescription
20 g/day (80 kcal)

Fat prescription
Calculate kcal intake from protein and carbohydrate: 288 + 80 = 368 kcal
Total kcal − kcal from protein and carbohydrate: 2000 − 368 = 1632 kcal
Calculate grams of fat: 1632/9 = 181 g

Daily prescription
The following figures should be seen as an approximate starting point:
kcal: 2000
Protein: 72 g, allowed freely (see Box 10.3)
Carbohydrate: 20 g = 4 × 5 g carbohydrate choices (see Box 10.5)
Fat: 181 g = 18 × 10 g fat choices (see Box 10.4)
Vitamin and mineral supplement

Box 10.2 Example meal plan based on calculation in Box 10.1 (18 fat choices and four carbohydrate choices daily).

Breakfast
Fat choices = 4, carbohydrate choices = 0
Scrambled egg: 3 fat choices as double cream, 1 fat choice as butter

Snack
Fat choices = 4, carbohydrate choices = 1
Strawberry smoothie: 4 fat choices as double cream, 1 carbohydrate choice as strawberry

Lunch
Fat choices = 5, carbohydrate choices = 1
Tuna mayonnaise: 5 fat choices as mayonnaise, 1 carbohydrate choice as tomato

Dinner
Fat choices = 5, carbohydrate choices = 2
Fried chicken with mushrooms and butternut squash and carrot mash: 2 fat choices as olive oil, 3 fat choices as double cream, 1 carbohydrate choice as carrot, 1 carbohydrate choice as butternut squash

Totals
Fat choices = 18
Carbohydrate choices = 4

Box 10.3 Example of selected high-protein foods allowed freely.

Keep it plain and simple – cook in oil, butter, or add double cream
Avoid processed meats, fish and eggs (e.g. sausages, fish fingers, scotch eggs and meat in sauces as they will have added carbohydrate in the form of breadcrumbs and flour)

- All meat including beef, pork, lamb, bacon, veal, ham, venison
- All poultry including chicken, turkey, duck, goose, poussin, quail, pheasant
- All fish including tuna (fresh or tinned in oil), salmon, sole, trout, sardines, herrings
- All shellfish including: prawns, crabmeat, squid, lobster, clams, oyster, mussels
- All eggs including scrambled, fried, poached, soft boiled, hard boiled, omelettes

---

Box 10.4 Example of selected 10-g fat choices.

Each of the following amounts is equal to one fat choice, or 10 g fat

- Butter: 3 teaspoons (1½ butter pats)
- Ghee: 3 teaspoons
- Sunflower margarine: 3 teaspoons
- Olive oil (or any pure vegetable oil): 1 dessertspoon
- Double cream (not Elmlea)*: 2 dessertspoons
- Mayonnaise*: 1 tablespoon (or 1 sachet)
- Calogen: 2 dessertspoons

Do *not* use any low-fat products such as low-fat spreads, reduced fat mayonnaise
Use only *full-fat* products

* These foods contain carbohydrate; check amount if using in large quantities.

However, the more liberal nature of this latter regimen meant that at times not enough fat was eaten to maintain weight or sustain ketosis and seizure control. In these circumstances it may be useful to increase the fat intake with a high-fat drink. This can be given as a prescribed amount of a fat emulsion with each meal using, for example, Calogen (Nutricia) added to tea or mixed with water and a low-carbohydrate flavouring. This follows a similar rationale to the Johns Hopkins use of a 300-mL Ketocal daily prescription to raise the diet's fat intake (Kossoff et al., 2011a). Experience shows that not all patients will need to be given extra fat; it is therefore better to increase the fat in the diet as necessary. Where there is a real concern about the amount of saturated fats in the diet, poly-unsaturated and monounsaturated fats can be encouraged as an alternative.

Carbohydrate

The daily dietary carbohydrate allowance is always prescribed for a MAD. Patients and their families, with the assistance of carbohydrate choice lists provided by the dietitian (Box 10.5), food labels and other manufacturer's information, translate this into meals and menus.

Box 10.5   Example of selected 5-g carbohydrate choices.

Each of the following amounts is equal to one carbohydrate choice, or 5 g carbohydrate. Free foods have a very low carbohydrate content and can be eaten freely

Apples (eating): ½ medium-sized apple
Apricots (raw): 1 medium fruit
Aubergine (cooked in oil): ½ medium aubergine
Avocado (flesh): ½ medium avocado
Banana: ¼ average size banana
Beansprouts (raw): 4 tablespoons
Beetroot (boiled): 1 small (whole)
Beetroot (pickled): 2 small (whole)
Blackberries (raw): ×20 fruits
Blueberries (raw): ×15 fruits
Broccoli (cooked): 4 tablespoons
Brussel sprouts (boiled): 4 sprouts
Butternut squash (boiled): 2 tablespoons
Cabbage/spring greens (boiled or raw): 4 tablespoons
Carrots (raw): 2 medium
Carrots (boiled): 2½ tablespoons
Cauliflower (raw or boiled): 4 tablespoons
Celery: free food
Clementine/satsuma: 1 fruit
Courgette (raw or cooked): 2 medium
Cucumber: free food
Curly kale (boiled/steamed): free food
French beans (cooked): 4 tablespoons
Grapefruit: ½ grapefruit
Gherkins (pickled): 2 large, or 4 small
Leeks (raw or cooked): 2 medium leeks (white part only)
Lettuce: free food
Mangetout (raw or cooked): 3 tablespoons
Mushrooms(raw): free food
Mustard and cress: free food
Onions (spring): 5 medium spring onions
Chopped onion: 2 tablespoons
Oranges: ½ medium orange
Pepper (red or yellow, raw or cooked): 5 rings
Plums: 1 fruit
Pumpkin (boiled): 4 tablespoons
Radish: free food
Raspberries: ×20
Rhubarb: free food
Runner beans (boiled): 4 tablespoons
Spinach (raw): free food
Strawberries: ×10
Swede (boiled): 4 tablespoons
Tomato (tinned or raw): 3 tablespoons (tinned) *or* 1 medium
Turnip (boiled): 4 tablespoons

Kossoff and his team recommend that all children on a MAD are started on 10 g of carbohydrate daily, as they found that using the higher amount of 20 g carbohydrate daily for the first 3 months compromised the future efficacy of the diet (Kossoff et al., 2007). However most of the centres surveyed from the UK and Ireland tended to be more cautious and start children on a higher amount of carbohydrate, ranging from 15 to 30 g daily; only one centre reported using the recommended 10 g. However, those centres which prescribed more initial carbohydrate all reported reducing this in response to the patient's level of ketosis and seizure control; these diet changes were made early in the diet initiation period and all within the first 3 months. Although this is in contrast to the protocol used in Kossoff et al.'s (2007) study where carbohydrate was maintained at 20 g daily for the whole 3-month period in the less-efficacious group, it is difficult to say whether the more cautious approach adopted by some centres in the UK and Ireland could have a detrimental effect on long-term efficacy. They certainly all reported that their patients became suitably ketotic and it is likely that prompt reduction of dietary carbohydrate means that the amounts of carbohydrate would be similar to those used at Johns Hopkins within 2–3 weeks of initiation.

The Johns Hopkins MAD protocol allows the prescribed carbohydrate to be eaten randomly through the day. As already discussed, this diet initially uses only 10 g of carbohydrate which is increased after a month. If an initial prescription uses a higher amount of carbohydrate, it is a sensible precaution to spread the carbohydrate evenly through the day, following the accepted practice of a classical or MCT KD. All the surveyed centres did recommend an even distribution of the prescribed carbohydrate allowance throughout the day.

In the first few weeks of starting the diet, if a larger amount of carbohydrate is prescribed, for example 30 g daily, this will allow the inclusion of small amounts of the higher-carbohydrate foods such as bread or pasta. However, as the diet is fine tuned, the carbohydrate prescription is usually reduced and is mainly provided by fruits and vegetables. The MAD does not include fibre as part of the carbohydrate allowance. Chapter 12 gives details on interpreting the carbohydrate and fibre contents listed on food labels.

Energy

On the MAD the patient's dietary energy intake need not be strictly controlled. An estimated energy requirement is useful so that advice can be given by the dietitian to the families and patients to ensure that energy intake is adequate. This estimated energy intake is only used for guidance, unlike the classical and MCT KD, where it has to be precisely calculated. When necessary, simple advice on how to adjust the energy intake can be given to the family. All the surveyed centres in the UK and Ireland weighed and measured their patients regularly to ensure that energy intake was adequate but not excessive.

Box 10.6   Example recipes for the MAD using food choice method

Eggs in the nest
2 eggs
Parmesan cheese to taste
3 teaspoons butter (1 fat choice)
2 dessertspoons double cream (1 fat choice)
Salt and pepper to taste

1 Preheat oven to 190 °C or gas mark 5.
2 Fill a baking tin halfway with boiling water.
3 Add butter to a small ovenproof dish and break eggs on top, and season.
4 Spoon over the double cream, and sprinkle with cheese.
5 Place the dish in the baking tin and cook for about 10 minutes until set.

Delicious strawberry smoothie
10 strawberries (1 carbohydrate choice)
4 dessertspoons double cream (2 fat choices)
Da Vinci syrup (strawberry flavour)
Water

1 Mix all the ingredients together in a blender.
2 If the smoothie is too thick, add some water.
3 Serve over ice.

Crunchy coleslaw
2 tablespoons raw shredded white cabbage (1/2 carbohydrate choice)
1 medium grated carrot (1/2 carbohydrate choice)
1 small spring onion
2 tablespoons mayonnaise (2 fat choices)
Lemon juice

Mix all the ingredients together.

Vitamin and mineral supplementation

As with the classical and MCT KD, a full vitamin and mineral supplement is required on the MAD (see Chapter 12). The diets should be monitored in the same way as a KD to ensure that they are nutritionally adequate (see Chapter 18).

Fluid intake

Fluid intake should be encouraged and at least normal requirements met.

Recipes

Using the food choice lists, recipes can be created (Box 10.6).

Conclusion

The food choice version of the MAD used in the UK and Ireland can be seen as both a relaxed version of the classical KD and modified version of the Johns Hopkins MAD. Principles relating to fat and protein content of the MAD used by some of the UK and Ireland centres are similar to those used in the USA. Further guidelines are needed on the initial carbohydrate prescription. An ideal may be to incorporate some of the principles of the low glycaemic index treatment, i.e. 10% of total daily energy taken as carbohydrate using carbohydrate foods with a low glycaemic index and allowing no more than 40–60 g of carbohydrate daily (see Chapter 11). This amount of prescribed carbohydrate would then be promptly reduced if necessary, in response to ketosis and seizure control, so avoiding the possible detrimental 3-month delay in such action.

Although there have been no formal studies as yet on the food choice method of administering MAD, it appears to offer the same potential to produce ketosis and therefore seizure control as the other types of dietary treatment, but is less rigid than the classical KD and therefore easier for patients to adhere to. As with all KD therapies it is essential that this should only be offered as a treatment by dietitians who have extensive experience in using these therapies for the treatment of epilepsy.

Acknowledgement

We are grateful to Jennifer Bosarge, Pediatric Dietitian, Johns Hopkins Hospital, Baltimore, USA for kindly reviewing this text.

References

Department of Health (1991) *Dietary Reference Values for Food Energy and Nutrients for the United Kingdom.* London: HMSO.

Kossoff, E.H., Krauss, G.L., McGrogan, J.R. and Freeman, J.M. (2003) Efficacy of the Atkins Diet as therapy for intractable epilepsy. *Neurology* **61**, 1789–1791.

Kossoff, E.H., McGrogan, J.R., Bluml, R.M., Pillas, D.J., Rubenstein, J.E. and Vining, E.P. (2006) A modified Atkins diet is effective for the treatment of intractable pediatric epilepsy. *Epilepsia* **47**, 421–424.

Kossoff, E.H., Turner, Z., Bluml, R.M., Pyzik, P.L. and Vining, E.P. (2007) A randomized crossover trial comparison of daily carbohydrate limits using the modified Atkins diet. *Epilepsy Behav* **10**, 432–436.

Kossoff, E.H., Dorward, J.L., Miranda, M.J., Wiemer-Kruel, A., Kang, H.C. and Kim, H.D. (2010) Will seizure control improve by switching from the Modified Atkins Diet to the traditional ketogenic diet? *Epilepsia* **51**, 2496–2499.

Kossoff, E.H., Freeman, J.M., Turner, Z. and Rubenstein, J.E. (2011a) *Ketogenic Diets: Treatments for Epilepsy and Other Disorders*, 5th edn. New York: Demos Medical Publishing.

Kossoff, E.H., Dorward, J.L., Turner, Z. and Pyzik, P.L. (2011b) Prospective study of the modified Atkins diet in combination with a ketogenic liquid supplement during the initial month. *J Child Neurol* **26**, 147–151.

Lord, K. and Magrath, G. (2010) Use of the ketogenic diet and dietary practices in the UK. *J Hum Nutr* **23**, 126–132.

Magrath, G., MacDonald, A. and Whitehouse, W. (2000) Dietary practices and use of the ketogenic diet in the UK. *Seizure* **9**, 128–130.

Chapter 11

The Low Glycaemic Index Treatment

Heidi H. Pfeifer

Massachusetts General Hospital, Boston, USA

Background and development

The treatment of epilepsy through dietary manipulation dates back to biblical times and to the texts of Hippocrates. Over time the therapy has evolved from pure fasting to the modern-day ketogenic diet (KD) protocol. Despite the liberalization of fluid and caloric intake, very few changes have been made to the original KD protocol, developed in the 1920s, and one that some institutions continue to use today (Kossoff et al., 2009).

In an effort to further advance the field of dietary therapy for epilepsy, the low glycaemic index treatment (LGIT) was developed in 2002 (Pfeifer and Thiele, 2005) as an alternative to the classical KD. Over the past 90 years, the efficacy of the KD has been well established; however, as demonstrated by the high dropout rate of those who initiate this dietary therapy, patient adherence remains a limiting factor to its clinical use (Henderson et al., 2006). Since the early 1990s, a renewed interest in the KD has driven an increased focus and attention on improving treatment initiation and maintenance for dietary protocols.

The exact mechanism of action of the KD currently remains unknown; the body of literature investigating the pathophyisologic mechanism underlying its anticonvulsant effect continues to grow. Specifically, it has been proven that systemic glucose levels in patients on the KD do remain quite stable even during prolonged periods of fasting (Valencia et al., 2002). Clinically, we have also observed a few specific cases where a dramatic increase in seizure activity directly followed the consumption of large amounts of carbohydrates, specifically those with a high glycaemic index (GI) value. It was the synthesis of these two observations that provided the initial inspiration for the development of the LGIT.

In 1981, Jenkins et al. reported that not only the quantity but also the type of carbohydrate ingested affects an individual's blood glucose response (Jenkins et al., 1981). This idea is captured by the GI of a given food and describes the

Dietary Treatment of Epilepsy: Practical Implementation of Ketogenic Therapy,
First Edition. Edited by Elizabeth Neal.
© 2012 John Wiley & Sons, Ltd. Published 2012 by John Wiley & Sons, Ltd.

degree to which it raises an individual's blood sugar relative to that of glucose. This value is calculated in the following way: 10 test subjects consume a quantity of a test food that contains 50 g of carbohydrate and their postprandial blood glucose is measured over a 2-hour period; this determines the area under the curve (AUC). On a separate occasion, the same 10 test subjects consume 50 g of glucose and their postprandial blood glucose AUC is again calculated over a 2-hour time interval. For each subject, the AUC of the test food is then divided by his or her AUC for glucose, and the average of these 10 quotients determines the GI of a given food (Brand-Miller et al., 2003). Unfortunately, GI data is not readily available for all foods due to the cost of this calculation.

Several variables contribute to the GI of a given food: level of acidity or type of fibre in a food, amount of processing and the foods with which it is paired. Generally, foods higher in fibre or acidity have a lower GI. Fibres such as pectin and guar gum can significantly reduce glycaemic response (Wolever and Jenkins, 2001). For example, a finely milled grain will have a lower fibre content and therefore a higher GI than that of the parent whole grain. Additionally, GI can also be lowered for a given food by pairing it with fat, as fat delays gastric emptying.

Dietary fibre consists of non-digestible carbohydrates that are fermented in the large intestine to short-chain fatty acids (butyrate, acetate, propionate) which are absorbed for energy. Although we know that the energy obtained from fibre is less that that obtained from carbohydrate (an estimated 1.5–2.5 kcal/g vs. 4 kcal/g), there are many influencing factors, including composition of food, dose of fibre, weight status of the individual and their digestive capability (Institute of Medicine, 2005). Therefore fibre is not subtracted out of a patient's goal daily carbohydrate intake.

Low GI diets have been used for years in the therapeutic treatment of many medical conditions, including diabetes, heart disease, obesity and polycystic ovary syndrome. The LGIT has been used to treat both seizures and polycystic ovary syndrome concurrently. In the setting of epilepsy, the LGIT limits total carbohydrate load to 40–60 g/day and limits carbohydrates to those with a GI of less than 50. The total daily carbohydrate parameter was derived from the physiologic threshold of 50 g/day, under which the body will begin to burn fat as the primary energy source.

Efficacy

The LGIT has been successful in treating both focal as well as generalized seizure types. Preliminary results on efficacy of the LGIT were first reported in 2005 in a retrospective review demonstrating that 73 % of patients had a 50 % or more reduction in seizure frequency compared with baseline, with one-third becoming seizure-free (Pfeifer and Thiele, 2005). More recently, a larger series indicated that 66 % of the patients had a 50 % or more reduction in seizure frequency compared with baseline after 1 year of treatment (Muzykewicz et al.,

> **Box 11.1   Case report of successful use of the LGIT**
>
> A 2½-year-old boy with tuberous sclerosis complex came to clinic for a second opinion. His history is significant for seizure onset that began at 6 months of age with infantile spasms. Within 4 days of onset he was treated with adrenocorticotropin (ACTH) and his spasms resolved. At the end of his ACTH treatment, approximately 8½ months of age, he began having a new seizure spell, which occurred three to four times a day, during which he would stop and have a scared look in his eyes sometimes with an irregular smile. In addition to the ACTH, his seizures remained refractory to levetiracetam, oxcarbazepine and zonisamide. During long-term EEG monitoring, a seizure focus was demonstrated and he was deemed a surgical candidate. Prior to surgery his parents wanted to make sure this was the correct decision.
>
> During this initial visit at Massachusetts General Hospital for Children, the LGIT was presented as a treatment option and the family was interested. Therefore they were educated on all aspects of providing the LGIT at home. Baseline blood levels and anthropometric measurements were obtained, and the family provided a 3-day food record, indicating that he consumed a daily average of 1230 kcal, 59 g protein (19%), 112 g carbohydrate (36%) and 62 g fat (45%). Based on this food record and calculations of his estimated needs, LGIT dietary goals for each day were provided to his family: 1200–1400 kcal, 40–60 g carbohydrates, 80–90 g fat, 80–90 g protein. After 2 weeks on the LGIT, he became seizure-free. After 1 year of dietary therapy, he sustained seizure freedom and was tapered off his two antiepileptic medications. He remained on the LGIT for another year, during which carbohydrates were slowly reintroduced. He now remains seizure-free, medication-free and is consuming a normal diet. Although he has been able to enjoy ice cream with the rest of the family, they continue to eat a majority of low-GI foods.

2009). Aligning with these findings, in a retrospective review of 15 patients, Coppola et al. (2011) found that 53% of patients had a 50% or more reduction in seizure frequency compared with baseline after 15 months of treatment.

We have also found the LGIT to be very effective in the treatment of patients with genetic disorders such as Angelman syndrome and tuberous sclerosis complex (Box 11.1). A prospective study found 67% had a greater than 90% reduction in seizure frequency compared with baseline after 4 months of treatment. All patients had improved EEG, with 75% showing complete resolution of epileptiform activity (Thibert et al., in preparation). Additionally, in a retrospective review of 15 patients with tuberous sclerosis complex, 47% had greater than 50% reduction in seizure frequency compared with baseline after 6 months of treatment (Larson et al., 2012). Treatment efficacy was found to positively correlate with lower blood glucose levels, but not with level of ketosis (Muzykewicz et al., 2009).

Initiation of an individualized treatment

When initiating a patient on the LGIT, baseline caloric intake should be evaluated. Close evaluation of a 3-day food record helps to establish the individual's daily caloric intake as well as the distribution of macronutrients and food habits.

The food record, in combination with energy requirement calculations by established means such as the Harris–Benedict equation, are used to determine the recommended energy goals. Additionally, anthropometric measurements are assessed so caloric intake can be adjusted for goals of weight increase or loss.

The recommended macronutrient distribution of the LGIT is 10% carbohydrate (40–60 g), 60% fat and approximately 30% protein. By comparison, the recommended distribution of energy intake for typical adults is 45–65% carbohydrate, 20–35% fat and 10–35% protein, with a similar range recommended for children (Institute of Medicine, 2005). The KD implements a ratio 3:1 or 4:1, grams of fat to grams of carbohydrate and protein. The LGIT implements a ratio of approximately 1:1. Because some patients consume much larger quantities of carbohydrates at baseline, initial goals may exceed 60 g/day but still result in a therapeutic change and reduction in seizure frequency. Individualized daily carbohydrate goals should therefore be set on a case-by-case basis and evaluated on an ongoing basis. The total daily carbohydrate allowance includes dietary fibre.

It is recommended that carbohydrate intake be evenly distributed throughout the day and always be paired with a protein and/or a fat source (e.g. a snack of half an apple with cheese) to decrease the overall GI of the meal or snack. Daily fluctuations in carbohydrate intake should also be limited to 5–10 g. An example LGIT calculation is shown in Box 11.2 and an example daily menu in Box 11.3.

Follow-up

To ensure safety when providing dietary treatment, routine follow-up with both a dietitian and a neurologist trained in this treatment modality is recommended. An ongoing and open dialogue between the clinician and patient and/or parents and caregivers is necessary to optimize treatment delivery. Formal clinic visits are recommended for 1 month after treatment is initiated, as well as every 3 months thereafter, and should include anthropometric measurements and a full haematological analysis of the following: complete blood count, electrolytes, liver, pancreatic and kidney function, lipid profile, carnitine, ketones, and vitamin and mineral levels. Finally, a urinalysis (including urine calcium/creatinine ratio) is routinely performed at each visit.

Fine tuning

To optimize the efficacy of the LGIT, adjustments may need to be made at any point during treatment. As no two patients are alike, responses to alterations may differ dramatically. It is important to keep the following in mind – calories, constipation, compliance and changes – as these are the factors that may need to be altered or addressed when working to improve seizure control.

Box 11.2   Example calculation of LGIT aiming for 1200 kcal daily

1 Multiply calories by 0.6 to provide 60% of calories from fat. Then divide that by 9 to determine grams of fat per day
   Calories × 0.6 = Calories from fat/9 = grams fat/day
   1200 × 0.6 = 720 calories from fat/9 = 80 g fat/day
2 Carbohydrates at 40–60 g/day provide 160–240 calories
3 Subtract calories from fat and carbohydrates from protein and then divide by 4 to determine grams of protein
   1200 − 720 = 480 − 160 = 320 calories from protein/4 = 80 g protein/day
   1200 − 720 = 480 − 240 = 240 calories from protein/4 = 60 g protein/day

Box 11.3   Sample daily LGIT menu

Case example goals
1200–1400 kcal/day
40–60 g carbohydrate
80–90 g fat
60–80 g protein

Breakfast
Scrambled egg with 2 eggs, 1 ounce* cheese, 1 teaspoon butter
Peach
Heavy cream, 1 ounce*
(Heavy cream is available in the USA and contains 36% fat)

Lunch
Roast beef sandwich comprising:
Low-carbohydrate pitta pocket, ½
Roast beef, 3 ounces*
Cheddar cheese, 1 ounce*
Horseradish mayonnaise, ½ tablespoon
Roasted red pepper, ½ cup
Heavy cream, 2 ounces*

Snack
Cheese chips, 1 ounce* (bake cheese on parchment paper until hard and crunchy)
Apple, ½

Dinner
Grilled chicken salad comprising:
Chicken breast, 4 ounces*
Mixed salad with lettuce, tomato and cucumber
Heavy cream, 2 ounces*
Blue cheese dressing, 1 tablespoon

* If using metric measures, 1 ounce = approximately 28 g.

- *Calories*. With an excessively high daily caloric intake, the metabolic response will tip towards storage of the fats consumed as opposed to mobilizing them for energy, resulting in weight gain. Conversely, inadequate caloric intake can result in metabolic stress and has the potential to exacerbate seizures.
- *Constipation*. Lack of regular bowel movements is a frequent side effect of the treatment, and ensuring that patients have regular bowel movements either daily or every other day is critical, as constipation can also exacerbate seizures. With many patients, laxative medication is used prophylactically.
- *Compliance*. Dietary compliance can clearly have a dramatic effect on the degree to which seizure control is obtained; however, deviation from dietary parameters is not always obvious to the parent or clinician. Small inadvertent increases in carbohydrates may result in a significantly higher overall daily intake. The following are two examples of common pitfalls in compliance: (i) because nuts and cream are so high in protein and fat, parents may forget to count their carbohydrate content towards the daily goals; and (ii) new medications or supplements might be introduced without realizing that they contain a significant amount of carbohydrates as additives. We therefore encourage families and caregivers to log daily intake through spreadsheets or computer web-based programs that include macronutrient data, so parents can easily monitor daily intake and compare these values with the treatment goals. An added benefit of this practice is that it can serve to aid clinicians when trying to identify specific trigger foods in the setting of increased seizure frequency.
- *Change*. Although somewhat ambiguous, this can refer to anything from purposeful treatment changes to changes in routine or sleep. There have been cases of increased waking during the night, exacerbating seizures, which was attributable to hunger and a need for caloric adjustment.

Micronutrient supplementation

Dietary restrictions required by the LGIT can affect an individual's micronutrient intake. To date, however, there have been no reported cases of significant deficiency in patients, as compared to the KD (see Chapter 18). Because the LGIT does limit the portion sizes of fruits, vegetables and dairy products, a complete multivitamin (with minerals) as well as a calcium supplement (with vitamin D) should be included in the dietary treatment to prevent micronutrient deficiency. Furthermore, ongoing review of food records in conjunction with routine monitoring of vitamin and mineral blood levels (see section on follow-up) is also recommended to ensure adequate intake of micronutrients.

In addition, vitamins and minerals can be supplemented by counselling patients and/or parents about the micronutrient content of some key foods that align well with the parameters of the LGIT. For example, Brazil nuts have high selenium content (1904 μg per 100 g), a low GI, and a macronutrient distribution compatible with the LGIT (12 g carbohydrate, 66 g fat and 14 g protein per 100 g) (National Institutes of Health, 2011).

Side effects

No significant side effects have been reported with the LGIT; however, as with any treatment, it is not without minor side effects. Slight weight loss is commonly seen during diet initiation. This is at least partly due to the diuretic effect of the carbohydrate reduction, but may also be due to an inadequate increase in the amount of protein and/or fat to compensate for the decrease in calories from carbohydrates. Metabolic acidosis may also occur as the body begins to metabolize fat as the primary energy source over carbohydrates, especially in the setting of concurrent treatment with a carbonic anhydrase inhibitor such as topiramate or zonisamide. As the symptoms of acidosis can mimic influenza-like symptoms such as nausea, vomiting and lethargy, it is commonly overlooked and sometimes viewed as intolerance to the diet. If a patient becomes acidotic, a potassium citrate solution is recommended (Paul et al., 2010). As previously discussed, constipation is common on the LGIT and therefore monitoring for bowel regularity is an integral part of treatment.

A commonly overlooked aspect of dietary treatment is the psychosocial impact of a highly restrictive diet. Not only do patients feel different from their peers because of their epilepsy, but now they also feel different due to their food restrictions. As many social occasions and holiday festivities revolve around food, it is important to empower patients and families with strategies on how to integrate treatment with these important events (see also Chapter 13).

Sick day management

During periods of illness, especially with increased vomiting or diarrhoea, it is important to maintain adequate hydration. As most oral electrolyte solutions contain dextrose, it is recommended to avoid them. Commercially available solutions may be 'sugar free' but still contain small amounts of carbohydrates. Good old-fashioned chicken broth can adequately provide the needed sodium (with minimum potassium) and is typically well tolerated. Additionally, in the setting of illness, it is critical to ensure that patients do not become overly acidotic, as this can perpetuate the vomiting cycle. Therefore, potassium citrate is supplemented at increased amounts above routine dosage. Intravenous hydration may be beneficial if clinicians or caregivers are unable to maintain adequate intake for the degree of output.

Diet discontinuation

Despite the liberalization of the LGIT over the KD and its proven efficacy, about 25–30% of patients will still need to discontinue the treatment due to difficulty with the restrictions (Muzykewicz et al., 2009; Coppola et al., 2011). Aside from being too restrictive, the diet is discontinued for a number of other reasons, including ineffectiveness, intercurrent illness and prolonged seizure freedom. When discontinued for an acute illness, weaning from the diet is done more abruptly. However, when weaning in the setting of long-term seizure control, the taper is typically done gradually over a period of months, increasing carbohydrates by 5–10 g increments to preserve seizure freedom. Avoidance of simple carbohydrates is recommended, especially in the initial stages.

Conclusion

The LGIT is now being used worldwide and plays an integral role as a treatment alternative for epilepsy. It is meeting a great clinical need in epilepsy care, as 36 % of seizure patients are considered pharmacoresistant, many of whom are not able to comply with the restrictions of the classical KD (Kwan and Brodie, 2000).

References

Brand-Miller, J., Wolever, T., Foster-Powell, K. and Colagiuri, S. (2003) *The New Glucose Revolution: The Authoritative Guide to the Glycemic Index, the Dietary Solution for Lifelong Health*, 5th edn. New York: Marlowe & Company.

Coppola, G., D'Aniello, A., Messana, T. et al. (2011) Low glycemic index diet in children and young adults with refractory epilepsy: first Italian experience. *Seizure* **20**, 526–528.

Henderson, C.B., Filloux, F.M., Alder, S.C., Lyon, J.L. and Caplin, D.A. (2006) Efficacy of the ketogenic diet as a treatment option for epilepsy: meta-analysis. *J Child Neurol* **21**, 193–198.

Institute of Medicine (2005) Dietary, functional, and total fiber. In: *Dietary Reference Intakes for Energy, Carbohydrates, Fiber, Fat, Fatty Acids, Cholesterol, Protein and Amino Acids*. Washington, DC: The National Academies Press.

Jenkins, D., Wolever, T., Talyor, R. et al. (1981) Glycemic index of foods: a physiological basis for carbohydrate exchange. *Am J Clin Nutr* **34**, 362–366.

Kossoff, E.H., Zupec-Kania, B.A., Amark, P.E. et al. (2009) Optimal clinical management of children receiving the ketogenic diet: recommendations of the International Ketogenic Diet Study Group. *Epilepsia* **50**, 304–317.

Kwan, P. and Brodie, M. (2000) Epilepsy after the first drug fails: substitution or add-on? *Seizure* **9**, 464–468.

Larson, A.M., Pfeifer, H.H. and Thiele, E. (2012) Low glycemic index treatment for epilepsy in tuberous sclerosis complex. *Epilepsy Res* **99**, 180–2.

Muzykewicz, D.A., Lyczkowski, D.A., Memon, N., Conant, K.D., Pfeifer, H.H. and Thiele, E.A. (2009) Efficacy, safety, and tolerability of the low glycemic index treatment in pediatric epilepsy. *Epilepsia* **50**, 1118–1126.

National Institutes of Health (2011) *Dietary Supplement Fact Sheet: Selenium*. Bethesda, MD: Office of Dietary Supplements, NIH.

Paul, E., Conant, K.D., Dunne, I.E. et al. (2010) Urolithiasis on the ketogenic diet with concurrent topiramate or zonisamide therapy. *Epilepsy Res* **90**, 151–156.

Pfeifer, H.H. and Thiele, E. (2005) Low glycemic index treatment: a liberalized ketogenic diet for treatment of intractable epilepsy. *Neurology* **65**, 1810–1812.

Valencia, I., Pfeifer, H. and Thiele, E.A. (2002) General anesthesia and the ketogenic diet: clinical experience in nine patients. *Epilepsia* **43**, 525–529.

Wolever, T. and Jenkins, D. (2001) Effect of dietary fiber and foods on carbohydrate metabolism. In: Spiller, G. (ed.) *Handbook of Dietary Fiber in Human Nutrition*, 3rd edn. Boca Raton, FL: CRC Press, pp. 321–362.

Chapter 12

Managing dietary treatment: further dietetic issues

Jan Chapple

Yorkhill Children's Hospital, Glasgow, UK

Further considerations when starting ketogenic diet (KD) therapy must include appropriate micronutrient supplementation, fluid intake, essential fatty acid requirements and any pre-existing food allergies or intolerances. These are discussed in this chapter. Details on other aspects of dietary implementation that parents or carers should be familiar with is also included.

Supplementation of vitamins, minerals and trace elements

The restrictive nature of KD therapies requires that all children are prescribed a vitamin and mineral supplement at diet initiation to prevent future deficiency. The carbohydrate-free supplement most commonly used in the UK is Phlexy-Vits (Nutricia), which is available in two preparations:

- powder: 30×7 g sachets per box
- tablets: 180 tablet pack, not recommended for children under 8 years.

This is available on prescription in the UK for use as a vitamin and mineral component of restricted therapeutic diets in children over 11 years. The suggested intake is one 7-g sachet per day or five tablets per day for children over 11 years and adults. The actual quantity should be determined by the dietitian considering age, weight and medical condition. Younger children will require smaller quantities to meet full nutritional requirements. These reduced quantities may be prescribed by the family doctor for children under the prescribing recommendations of 11 years; this must be requested individually on a named patient basis. An alternative has recently been developed; FruitiVits (Vitaflo) is an orange-flavoured, palatable, low-carbohydrate powdered vitamin, mineral and trace

Dietary Treatment of Epilepsy: Practical Implementation of Ketogenic Therapy,
First Edition. Edited by Elizabeth Neal.

element supplement that can be prescribed in the UK for use in restrictive therapeutic diets for children aged 3–10 years. The 6 g sachet of powder dissolves in 60 mL water.

Intake of vitamin and mineral preparations should be closely monitored. Compliance can often be poor due to tolerability of the product. There have been recent developments in commercially available sugar-free vitamin and mineral preparations for children, and these may be more acceptable than preparations available on prescription. If alternative vitamin and mineral supplements are used that do not provide full nutritional requirements, additional individual supplements are likely to be required. Children on the medium-chain triglyceride (MCT) KD may not need the amount of calcium supplement given with the classical KD, due to the incorporation of more milk and dairy products; this should be assessed individually. The modified Atkins diet (MAD) and low glycaemic index treatment (LGIT) are more liberal than the KD and may require a reduced level of supplementation. Current practice varies: some centres supplement to full requirements and other to only half requirements.

Blood nutrient levels should be monitored (see Chapter 18) and individual deficiencies may require additional supplementation. The carbohydrate content of each supplement preparation should be considered. It is suggested that actual nutrient intake from all diets is analysed annually to determine optimal supplement level.

Essential fatty acids

Essential fatty acids (EFA) have received significant attention in relation to improved neurological function and ability and so it is understandable that parents are keen to ensure adequate intake of these nutrients. There are two types of EFA, omega-3 and omega-6. Typical Western diets tend to contain higher levels of omega-6 fatty acids than recommended, and healthy eating guidelines recommend lowering omega-6 intake and increasing omega-3, by reducing intake of processed foods, including oily fish in the diet, and replacing some of the commonly used vegetable oils with oils higher in omega-3 or with olive oil. All KD therapies must supply sufficient amounts of EFA, and a good balance between omega-3 and omega-6 fatty acids can be achieved by varying the oil source where possible. For those using large amounts of polyunsaturated vegetable oils, a small amount (2–3 mL) of omega-3 rich oil can be added to the diet daily, using oil such as flaxseed, linseed, hempseed or walnut. This is also of importance for children following the MCT KD, especially if receiving a large percentage of their energy from the MCT source, to ensure that adequate EFA are provided. Within the constraints of the prescribed diet, regular omega-3 food sources should be encouraged, such as oily fish and dark green vegetables. The use of an EFA-containing prescribed fat supplement and Ketocal (Nutricia) will also improve intake. Some commercially available EFA products also contain evening primrose oil, which was once implicated as causing or increasing seizures although this has since been discredited (Puri, 2007) and contraindications for the use of evening primrose oil in epilepsy have been removed from all medical formularies.

If using omega-3 rich oils as a supplement, this should be limited to the small amounts already mentioned to avoid any risks from high doses, and the extra calories may need to be included into the dietary prescription. There are also some concerns over the high level of fat-soluble vitamins in all EFA-rich oils, in particular vitamins A and E. Both of these vitamins are constituents of the pre-scribed vitamin and mineral supplement. In view of the risk of toxicity, levels of these vitamins should be monitored regularly.

Free foods, sweeteners and sugar alcohols

Free foods include sugar-free drinks such as water, diet fizzy drinks and squashes and some spices, stocks and essences to be used in cooking. A few centres allow some free fruit and vegetables which have minimal amounts of carbohydrate. These foods can aid compliance by improving the palatability of meals and the additional vegetables can reduce symptoms of constipation. Although their carbohydrate content is limited, they should be reduced or removed if ketosis and/or seizure control is poor.

Saccharin- and aspartame-based sweeteners are recommended. Although there are some suggestions that aspartame may trigger seizures (Wurtman, 1985; Camfield et al., 1992), other studies do not support this (Shaywitz et al., 1994; Rowan et al., 1995) and most children continue to use it without a problem. Liquid sweeteners mix easily into meals and baking and can usually be ordered by local pharmacies if not in stock (see Chapter 13).

Sugar alcohols are a hydrogenated form of carbohydrate. Examples are arabitol, erythritol, glycerol, isomalt, actitol, maltitol, mannitol, sorbitol and xylitol. They are not as sweet as some synthetic sweeteners and are used in conjunction with them to mask their unpleasant aftertaste. They are usually incompletely absorbed into the bloodstream from the small intestine which results in a smaller change in blood glucose than sucrose; however they do still yield some energy (Beaugerie et al., 1997) and are not routinely recommended for use when following KD treatments. Diabetic products and some 'low carb' foods are also unsuitable for use in the KD as they contain sugar alcohols and bulk sweeteners; although the latter are often included in the Atkins diet for weight loss, they are generally not suitable for use in the MAD or LGIT for the above reasons. There are some other ingredients found in foods and medicines that are plant based but which do not contain absorbable carbohydrate so can be included. Examples are cellulose, carboxymethylcellulose, hydroxymethylcel-lulose and microcrystalline cellulose.

Table 12.1   Guidelines for using food label information while on a ketogenic dietary treatment for epilepsy.

Nutrient information listed on label	Presentation of nutrient values	
	Per 100 g	Per pack/serving
Fat:	Yes	No
of which saturated fat	No	No
Protein:	Yes	No
Carbohydrate:	Yes	No
of which sugar	No	No
Fibre:	No	No

Reading labels

Flexibility and variety are essential to improve compliance with the dietary treatments. Families should be instructed on how to read food labels accurately, allowing them to use new products and manipulate meals to suit products which are available. Products should be re-checked regularly as compositions may change over time due to manufacturing changes. Parents or carers should be directed to look only at the macronutrients provided by 100 g of product (Table 12.1).

In Europe there is often confusion about the term 'net carbs', used in many Atkins and MAD guides originating from the USA. This refers to the total carbohydrate content after the fibre has been subtracted. European nutrition labels always list fibre separately rather than as part of a total carbohydrate figure so the 'carbohydrate' figure stated on a European product label is the value that should be used in a calculation, and is equivalent to the 'net carbs' referred to in the USA guides.

Fluids

Traditionally fluid was restricted to 90% of requirements. As there is no scientific evidence to support this, fluid restriction beyond normal amounts is not currently recommended (Vaisleib et al., 2004). Low-carbohydrate diets have a diuretic effect and unlike a normal diet the contribution of fluid from the restricted volume of foods in the dietary treatment is minimal. It is essential to ensure an adequate fluid intake where possible as renal stones may be a side effect (see Chapter 18). Parents should be advised on appropriate fluid intake for age and weight; advice should be given if intake is excessive or inadequate. Excess intake can dilute urine ketone levels and dehydration can cause an artificially high reading.

Special occasions

Special occasions should not be avoided by children on KD treatments. Many parents are skilled in developing ketogenic-friendly meals and snacks to suit most occasions. Children can attend parties, taking their own party bag, or go out to dinner taking a special diet meal to be heated up at the venue. Families have successfully gone on holiday in the UK and abroad; some have taken a laptop with a computer program such as Electronic Ketogenic Manager (EKM) to allow them to enter local product data and amend meals to suit ingredients available. Customs letters may be required to allow those travelling abroad to carry prescribed dietary products or special preprepared meals onto the aircraft. Parents are advised to contact their travel company direct for advice.

Food allergy or intolerance

It is possible to follow a KD treatment in addition to excluding specific food groups as a result of allergy or intolerance (see Box 12.1 for an example meal plan). However, combining the food restrictions of both regimens can reduce choice and hinder compliance. Common childhood allergies or intolerances such as milk, egg and nuts can be catered for successfully but children with multiple allergies or intolerances may not be appropriate candidates for a dietary treatment.

Ketocal (Nutricia) contains milk protein, and therefore for children with milk allergy or intolerance a milk-free alternative should be calculated for use as a ketogenic drink or enteral feed during periods of illness. The child's current formula or milk alternative could be used as a base with added fat, carbohydrate and protein modules as needed. If using as an enteral feed, then the addition of vitamins, minerals, trace elements and electrolytes may be needed to ensure nutritional adequacy (see Chapter 14).

Topical creams and toothpaste

Some parents have reported changes in ketone levels that can only be attributed to the use of creams or lotions such as sun cream, moisturizers and nappy creams. They report no dietary deviation or other external factors such as medicines or illness which could account for the changes seen. However, paediatric dermatologist colleagues report that it is highly unlikely that the carbohydrates contained in such products would be absorbed via the skin. Most creams and lotions can be used without effect; if problems persist it should be ensured that the product is not being consumed orally or the skin licked. Medicines information should be consulted for specific product advice if appropriate.

It is often recommended that all children following a KD or other similar dietary regimens should use baking soda toothpaste as an alternative as this has

Box 12.1   Example of milk-free classical ketogenic diet

- Female, 7 years, weight 29 kg
- Classical diet at 3:1 ratio, requirements 1980 kcal/day and 29 g protein per day
- Four meals, each providing: 47.90 g fat, 7.25 g protein, 8.72 g carbohydrate

Breakfast

		Carbohydrate (g)	Fat (g)	Protein (g)
Eggs, chicken, whole, raw	46.0 g	5.15	5.75	0.00
Calogen (Nutricia)	40.0 g	20.00	0.00	0.00
Olive oil	15.0 g	14.98	0.00	0.00
Tomatoes, raw	20.0 g	0.06	0.14	0.62
White bread, sliced	18.0 g	0.29	1.42	8.30
Pure sunflower spread	11.0 g	7.37	0.00	0.00
Totals		47.85	7.31	8.92

Lunch

		Carbohydrate (g)	Fat (g)	Protein (g)
Pure sunflower spread	14.0 g	9.38	0.00	0.00
Mayonnaise, retail	30.0 g	22.68	0.33	0.51
Tuna, canned in brine, drained	22.0 g	0.13	5.17	0.00
Wholemeal rolls	18.0 g	0.59	1.87	8.30
Calogen (Nutricia)	30.0 g	15.00	0.00	0.00
Totals		47.78	7.37	8.81

Evening meal

		Carbohydrate (g)	Fat (g)	Protein (g)
Chicken, light meat, raw	22.0 g	0.24	5.28	0.00
Carrots, young, raw	13.0 g	0.07	0.09	0.78
Beansprouts, mung, raw	15.0 g	0.07	0.44	0.60
Noodles, egg, raw	9.0 g	0.74	1.09	6.45
Vegetable oil, blended, average	34.0 g	33.97	0.00	0.00
Alpro single cream	20.0 g	2.10	0.42	0.90
Calogen (Nutricia)	21.0 g	10.50	0.00	0.00
Totals		47.69	7.32	8.73

Supper

		Carbohydrate (g)	Fat (g)	Protein (g)
Calogen (Nutricia)	84.0 g	42.00	0.00	0.00
Alpro soya unsweetened milk	165.0 g	2.97	5.44	0.33
Cocoa powder	7.0 g	1.52	1.30	0.81
Gingernuts	10.0 g	1.58	0.50	7.50
Totals		48.07	7.24	8.64

a reduced quantity of carbohydrate. However, this can be too strong for children and there are limited products which are suited to the lower fluoride levels required for younger children. Natural, sugar and sweetener-free children's toothpaste brands could be used as alternatives, for example Tom's of Maine. Dental hygiene is essential; if necessary children can continue with their existing toothpaste, ensuring the quantity used is not excessive and residue is expelled and not swallowed.

Concluding comment

Attention to the issues discussed in this chapter as part of the dietary implementation process will help establish a smooth transition onto KD therapy. Further practical advice, given from a parent's perspective, is included in Chapter 13.

References

Beaugerie, L., Flourié, B., Pernet, P., Achour, L., Franchisseur, C. and Rambaud, J.C. (1997) Glucose does not facilitate the absorption of sorbitol perfused in situ in the human small intestine. *J Nutr* **127**, 341–344.

Camfield, P.R., Camfield, C.S., Dooley, J.M., Gordon, K., Jollymore, S. and Weaver, D.F. (1992) Aspartame exacerbates EEG spike-wave discharge in children with generalized absence epilepsy: a double blind controlled study. *Neurology* **42**, 1000–1003.

Puri, B.K. (2007) The safety of evening primrose oil in epilepsy. *Prostaglandins Leukot Essent Fatty Acids* **77**, 101–103.

Rowan, A.J., Shaywitz, B.A., Tuchman, L., French, J.A., Luciano, D. and Sullivan, C.M (1995) Aspartame and seizure susceptibility: results of a clinical study in reportedly sensitive individuals. *Epilepsia* **36**, 270–275.

Shaywitz, B.A., Anderson, G.M., Novotny, E.J., Ebersole, J.S., Sullivan, C.M. and Gillespie, S.M. (1994) Aspartame has no effect on seizures or epileptiform discharges in epileptic children. *Ann Neurol* **35**, 98–103.

Vaisleib, I.I., Buchalter, J.R. and Zupanc, M.L. (2004) Ketogenic diet: outpatient initiation, without fluid or caloric restrictions. *Pediatr Neurol* **31**, 198–202.

Wurtman, R.J. (1985) Aspartame: possible effect on seizure susceptibility. *Lancet* **ii**, 1060.

Chapter 13

Managing dietary treatment: a parent's perspective

Emma Williams

Matthew's Friends Charity and Clinics, Lingfield, UK

Background: parental fears and anxieties

Parenting a child with intractable epilepsy involves a roller coaster of emotions, including fear, guilt, grief, anxiety, anger, and feeling overwhelmed and terrified. Many families have gone through hell and back by the time they actually get to the point of discussing dietary treatment and going forward with it. Just the fact of being referred for a ketogenic diet (KD) therapy means that medication has not worked in controlling their child's seizures so the families are already very familiar with disappointment and family life has changed dramatically from what they thought it was going to be like; it is very much like a grieving process.

In some respects the food they are able to feed their child becomes even more important, especially if it is the one way that the parents can show their love or the nurturing side of things – giving the child their favourite things to eat and treats such as chocolate or sweets after particularly bad episodes of seizures are a way of trying to 'make things better' for the child – to then ask the families to take that away as well can sometimes be extremely distressing for them. Children also become fixated on things and food can be one of the major ones, so making dietary changes can become very frightening for the family who could be under an immense amount of stress at home. If a child is severely disabled with complex seizures there is often pressure financially as one parent may have to stop working to be the main carer; this may also have an impact on the amount of time that they can spend with any siblings. To then add to this stress by asking parents to do a restrictive diet can invoke a look of panic in their faces and one that I have seen quite often in the various clinics I have sat in on over the years.

Dietary Treatment of Epilepsy: Practical Implementation of Ketogenic Therapy,
First Edition. Edited by Elizabeth Neal.

Although a dietary treatment is yet more responsibility for the parents, at the same time it can give hope: a chance to get more control back and try something different from medications with their potential side effects. The family will know that it could be the only treatment that works for their child, yet feel guilty for secretly not actually *wanting* a diet because of the extra work, stress and responsibility it may involve. Up to this point in their child's treatment a family usually just follows instructions on medication; now much of the success of the dietary treatment working is based on what *they* do and *how* they do it.

These conflicting thoughts can be overwhelming for families and often lead to sleepless nights. In some instances working towards a more positive frame of mind can be the biggest obstacle for the ketogenic team to overcome. Some families will need 'baby steps' towards building their own confidence up and will need to make very small changes to their child's diet, sometimes over the course of weeks. Although this may seem time-consuming, especially for a treatment where the outcome is uncertain, greater success is achieved with the diet if you have a committed and confident family. Taking the time to talk through anxieties will be a great help to the families so they can actually voice their concerns.

Preparation for the diet and getting started: advice for the family

Commit for 3 months

Three months is not a long period of time and will be necessary to build the diet up to the level it needs to be and allow for fine tuning. It is a good idea for the family to clear as much as they can at home and try to make sure that they give the diet 100%. It is usually the case that if there is to be any improvement using the diet, it will be seen within the first 3 months. If there is no change whatsoever either in seizure control or the day-to-day well-being, then it is unlikely (although not always the case – each person must be evaluated individually) that the diet is the appropriate treatment.

If at the end of 3 months things have not gone well and sadly the diet has not worked, at least the family will know that they did their very best and did everything correctly; they can then move on from it and try a different treatment.

What do they consider failure or success in using the diet?

This should be discussed with the family who must be really honest as to what their expectations are. Deep down, they all hope for complete seizure control, no medications and an end to the nightmare, and for some that dream *will* come true. For those who have children with very difficult to control epilepsy who have gone through years of medication, seizures and hospital visits, it may be wise to

---

Box 13.1   The importance of family support

"I remember having the family over for dinner in the early days of the diet and my mum expressing how sorry she was for Matthew because he couldn't have the treacle sponge pudding we were all having, so I asked her if she would prefer Matthew to go back to having hundreds of seizures all the time and the fact that he couldn't actually have participated at sitting at the dinner table with the family before the diet. Obviously she was horrified at that prospect and it was the last thing she wanted for her grandson but she just hadn't thought it through before she said anything. Matthew was more than happy tucking into his own pudding I hasten to add!"

---

lower expectations at first and take it a step at a time. Adults who have had seizures since childhood and are on cocktails of medications may take longer to see benefit but the diet can make them feel so much better, improve their recovery time from seizures and improve their quality of life. It is important to be realistic, and focus on *all* the possible benefits of the diet. Keeping a daily diary might be useful to track changes.

Talk to everyone

The dietary treatment should be discussed with all the family, who should be given relevant information. It is important to have as many people on board especially in the beginning. Siblings must understand that they won't be able to share their sweets with their brother or sister. Close family friends also need to be made aware. The more support available, the better the chances of success. It is quite usual to be met with sympathy or pity and for the focus to immediately be on the negative (Box 13.1), but when discussing the diet with others, the possible positive outcomes should be focused on, such as seizure reduction or even freedom, improved quality of life, reduction of medications and the taking back of some control for a child's treatment which can be very empowering.

Shopping for the diet

Before starting dietary treatment stock up on the basic essentials that will be needed (Box 13.2). As confidence grows on the diet, the shopping list can be expanded to include a wider variety of ingredients (Box 13.3).

Cream can be used in many ketogenic recipes. If using a supermarket's own brand, check the label to ensure values are similar to those used to calculate the recipes. Clotted cream is another good option being very high in fat. Cream cheese is excellent as a sauce (just need to water it down slightly) and can add flavour to a meal. The 'light' versions should not be used, but always full fat or 'original' and if buying the shop's own brands read the labels to make sure that they are similar to the branded products.

Box 13.2   Basic shopping list for KD therapy

Butter
Double cream
Mayonnaise
Eggs
Bacon
Mature cheddar cheese: will give more flavour
Oil: vegetable/olive oil/coconut oil
Cocoa
Sugar-free jelly
Sweeteners: Hermesetas liquid or tablets
Squash/water/diet fizzy drinks
Chicken
Beef mince
Mushrooms: absorb fat very well and also good on quantity
Vegetables: frozen or fresh
Salad vegetables
Mixed herbs and garlic powder

Box 13.3   Expanded shopping list for KD therapy

Tuna in oil
Coconut oil
Ground almonds
Brazil nuts
Cream cheese
Peanut butter
DaVinci syrups
Rhubarb
Cranberries
Blueberries
Chinese leaf
Curly kale
Duck
Quorn
Shirataki noodles

Duck is a good meat to include because it is high in fat; buying just the legs in a small pack is recommended so it doesn't end up being too expensive. Quorn mince or pieces are an excellent protein replacement. The mince is particularly useful as it appears a larger quantity when you weigh it out compared to its meat counterpart. It is best used in strongly flavoured recipes. Nuts are excellent for making cookies and cakes and are also good for snacks if appropriate.

Coconut oil is a natural source of medium-chain triglyceride (MCT) that can be used on the classical and MCT KDs. It is available from most supermarkets and is great for ketogenic baking and frying. As coconut oil can increase ketosis it should only be used by a family after discussion with the dietitian.

Tips for low-carbohydrate meals

- High-carbohydrate fruits and vegetables such as carrots and grapes can be replaced with low-carbohydrate versions. Salad vegetables are the lowest in carbohydrate: lettuce leaves can be used instead of wraps and Chinese leaf is great in salads and stir fry. Always try to go for berries as a fruit as they are low in carbohydrate. Cranberries, rhubarb and blueberries are great stewed with some sweetener as a pudding or put in a baked egg custard or used with ketogenic pancakes. Potatoes always seem to be the one item that is most missed on KD therapies. For stricter versions of the diet then celeriac (also known as celery root) can be used in every way that you would normally use potatoes. This low-carbohydrate vegetable has been a life saver for some families and can make great crisps, chips, roast and mashed potato substitutes.
- Shirataki noodles or 'miracle noodles' are thin, long, translucent noodles made from very fine strands of a gelatinous substance called glucomannan, which is taken from the Devil's tongue plant (Japanese yam). Their texture is slightly rubbery and they don't have a flavour of their own, but pick up the flavour of the other ingredients in the dish in which they are simmered so are good with highly flavoured sauces. They are exceptionally low in carbohydrate, high in fibre and can be used to replace pasta and rice. They are packaged in water and should be drained and rinsed thoroughly before use. Available from www.locarbmegastore.com.
- Replace ordinary flour with low-carbohydrate alternatives such as soya flour, ground almonds or coconut flour to make ketogenic cakes and biscuits, for example blueberry muffins and MCT flapjacks. Recipes are available at www.matthewsfriends.org. The product Ketocal (Nutricia), available on prescription in the UK for use with KD therapy, can also be used to make ketogenic bread, pastry, pizza bases, scones and crumbles, as well as in cake and biscuit recipes.
- Hermesetas liquid is a useful sweetener that can be used in cooking and baking. In the UK it is available, or can be ordered, from pharmacies. An alternative is to use sweetener tablets dissolved in some boiling water; this can then be stored in the fridge and used as a liquid sweetener when required.
- DaVinci syrups come in many different varieties and can be used for baking. They are very useful as they sweeten and flavour at the same time. Available from www.locarbmegastore.com.
- Always read the labels and beware of hidden carbohydrate sources (Box 13.4). If something says 'sugar free' it doesn't necessarily mean it is carbohydrate free.

Eating away from home

Planning ahead for occasions and meals out can make all the difference. The family must focus on what *can* be included rather than what cannot, and remember that when socializing with friends and having a good time the food becomes

Box 13.4 An item with one of these ingredients on the label contains some carbohydrate and may need to be avoided or the carbohydrate calculated into the diet

Cereal	Polysaccharide
Corn starch	Dextrose
Corn sweetener	Fructose
Corn syrup	Galactose
Corn syrup solids	Glucose
Flour	Lactose
Fruit extract	Levulose
High fructose corn syrup	Maltose
Hydrogenated starch hydrolysate	Mannose
Invert syrup	Polydextrose
Malt sugar	Sucrose
Molasses	Xylose
Sorghum	Glycerol
Starch	Maltodextrin
Sugar	Dextrin
Sugarcane	Glycerine
Syrup	Sorbitol
Disaccharide	Xylitol
Monosaccharide	Mannitol

Box 13.5 Basic ideas for ketogenic eating out

- Choose plain meats with no coatings such as breadcrumbs or batters.
- Use salad-type vegetables where possible or take own recommended list of vegetables and scales if necessary.
- Ask for oil-based dressings or extra butter or mayonnaise with the meal.
- Take own pudding (e.g. sugar-free jelly or low-carbohydrate berries) and ask for additional cream.
- Diet drinks and/or water with meals.
- Black coffee or tea (with cream and sweetener added if wished).
- Fruit or herbal unsweetened teas.

secondary. A phone call beforehand may help. Basic ideas are given in Box 13.5. Barbecues are easy as mostly meat and salads. Buffets are also fairly simple as there is usually a mix of foods to choose from; however, if it is a sandwich tea it might be worthwhile packing a ketogenic salad or 'packed' supper and just adding allowed food to it from the buffet table. Picnics are easy if cold meats, cheeses and salads are used.

Grill restaurants such as Harvester and Beefeater are very good options for ketogenic eating out, with choices of cooked plain meats and salad bars. Care should be taken with gravy and sauces as they have thickening agents in them. For example, instead of having a steak with sauce on, ask for a steak with some cheese on if something extra is wanted. Fast food restaurants frequently provide nutritional information on their websites. Avoid fries or chips, battered or breaded fish or meats and bread or burger buns. Eating out at an Indian restaurant can be difficult to monitor, but curries can easily be incorporated into daily menus using dried curry spices, double cream and/or creamed coconut with meat or fish. Chinese food is also a challenge, and best homemade, for example stir fry from very low carbohydrate vegetables or roasted crispy duck or pork. Chinese five spice, soy sauce or fish sauce can be used to flavour vegetables.

Solving everyday problems

What happens if the child is at school and spills their lunch?

1   If family live near, then bring another meal in.
2   Keep an emergency meal in the school freezer such as an all-in-one ketogenic muffin or quiche. A ketogenic meal replacement drink could also be kept at school or the recipe and ingredients for one.
3   If neither of the above is possible, the parents or carer should be telephoned to discuss any options the school kitchen has available. A meal could be put together using protein, fat and small amounts of vegetables.

What happens if the child eats somebody else's food?

1   Remove as much of the offending article as possible as safely as possible.
2   If carbohydrates have been taken, try giving some fat to try to balance this out, for example Calogen or Liquigen (both Nutricia) or oil or butter.
3   The calories of the next meal could be reduced or a snack omitted.
4   Ketones and blood glucose should ideally be checked before any action is taken as it may be that the indiscretion will only have a transitory effect.
5   In some cases this is discovered later and there may be nothing that can be done; it should be ensured that the family has emergency antiepileptic medications in the house and that the diet is very accurate for next few days.

What happens if the child gets upset at mealtimes and refuses to eat?

1   Avoid the child picking up on any family anxiety around eating and finishing the food. Put food in front of the child and let them get on with it or if feeding your child, then try a spoonful – if they refuse take it away and carry on doing other things, leaving a longer gap in between trying or giving the child something to distract them from the plate of food. The meal may have to be taken away and then offered again when the child is hungry or a ketogenic meal replacement drink used instead.

2 Change the pattern and the meal times if necessary. Feed children somewhere other than the table, a picnic in the garden (weather permitting) for instance. Use distraction methods, such as letting them have their meal in front of the TV. Some families may not like the idea but it will be helpful if a battle is avoided.

3 If children see their family eating something different this can be the cause of stress and guilt for parents. Families should be encouraged to eat similar things to the child – everyday family meals can easily be adapted for ketogenic foods, for example substituting roast celeriac instead of roast potatoes.

What happens if the child isn't hungry and won't finish their meals?

1 The dietitian can assess overall calorie intake and consider whether meals can be made smaller.

2 Change from three big meals a day to four smaller ones.

3 Reduce or remove snacks.

4 Check ketone levels. If the child routinely doesn't want to eat when their ketones are at a good or high level, then the level of ketosis may need to be lowered.

What happens if the child no longer likes the ketogenic meals they used to like?

1 Avoid particular disliked meals for a while and reintroduce after a break of a couple of weeks.

2 Try to make meals look different; a couple of drops of food colouring may help in some instances!

Chapter 14

Enteral feeding

Jan Chapple

Yorkhill Children's Hospital, Glasgow, UK

The ketogenic diet (KD) can be easily delivered as an enteral feed, i.e. through a tube directly into the stomach, duodenum or jejunum. The most commonly used route of feeding is to the stomach, using a gastrostomy or nasogastric tube. Efficacy of the diet in this form is high (Kossoff et al., 2004; Hosain et al., 2005) and as would be expected there is an increase in compliance over ketogenic meals. It is also suggested that calculating the prescription of a ketogenic enteral feed is simpler for dietitians and requires less education for families or patients. Due to ease of delivery ketosis can be easily achieved and errors are less common. However, where possible, oral ability should not be compromised; those who are able to eat should not be prevented from doing so simply for the above reasons.

There are two situations where a ketogenic enteral feed is useful: for existing enterally fed patients who are to be initiated on a KD, and for patients already established on a KD therapy who subsequently require enteral feeding. Both situations are considered separately during this chapter.

The classical KD is the preferred option for existing enterally fed children. Ketocal 4:1 (Nutricia) is a high-fat, low-carbohydrate, nutritionally complete powder formula for the dietary management of intractable epilepsy in children over the age of 1 year. Formulated to induce and maintain ketosis, it is based on the classical 4:1 ratio. It is available in neutral or vanilla flavour and has a recommended concentration of 20 g per 100 mL which yields a 1.5 kcal/mL feed. Ketocal multifibre LQ (Nutricia) is a newly launched liquid feed preparation which is currently only available in vanilla flavour. This ready-to-feed 4:1 ketogenic formulation provides 150 kcal, 3.09 g protein, 0.61 g carbohydrate, 14.8 g fat and 1.12 g fibre per 100 mL. It can provide complete nutritional support or supplemental feeding from 1 to 10 years of age, and may be used for supplemental feeding over the age of 10 years.

Ketocal products must only be used under strict medical supervision and patients should be monitored closely for hypoglycaemia, renal stones, adequate growth and hyperlipidaemia (see Chapter 18). Ketocal is available on prescription in the UK and is dispensed via the Nutricia Homeward home delivery system.

Calculating ketogenic enteral feeds for existing enteral feeders

Some centres use Ketocal prepared as the manufacturers suggest to a 4:1 ratio, providing the appropriate volume to meet the child's specific energy requirements. Other centres calculate the actual diet prescription and modify Ketocal by adding additional fat and carbohydrate modules to meet the exact diet prescription.

If current growth and hydration is adequate, then the energy prescription and fluid allowance of the current enteral feed is a good starting point. Protein requirement should be determined, a general guideline being 1 g/kg daily for older children and 1.5 g/kg daily for rapidly growing younger children. The appropriate diet ratio should then be selected and the KD prescription calculated (see Chapter 8); this will then be translated into an enteral feed rather than meals (see example in Box 14.1).

Transition to ketogenic enteral feed from an existing enteral feed

There are two suggested methods of transition: to introduce the ketogenic feed as a percentage of the existing enteral feed, or to introduce full ketogenic feeds at a reduced ketogenic ratio.

Introducing ketogenic feeds as a percentage of existing enteral feeds

If using this method only the desired ratio of ketogenic enteral feed needs to be calculated as this would be mixed with the existing enteral feed to produce a lower ratio for initiation. Difficulty may arise if ketones are consistently high when still on a mixture of existing enteral feed and ketogenic feed. Table 14.1 provides details of this method.

Introducing full ketogenic feeds at a reduced ratio

Introducing full ketogenic feeds at a reduced ratio requires more calculations but allows the ratio to be gradually increased, stopping when optimal ketone levels are achieved. Table 14.2 provides details of this method, and a worked example

Box 14.1   Example calculation of a classical KD enteral feed

Prescription
- 18-month-old boy, weight 10.2 kg, height 77.6 cm
- On current feed of 1200 kcal/day, as 800 mL of 1.5 kcal/mL feed given as bolus feeds of 200 mL ×4 via pump at 200 mL/hour every 4 hours. Additional water is given as 25 mL flush before and after feed, providing a total fluid volume of 1000 mL/day.
- Protein requirement 1.5 g/kg daily = 10.2 kg × 1.5 g = 15.3 g/day
- Ratio selected 3 : 1
- Continue 1200 kcal/day
- Using dietary unit method (see Chapter 8), total enteral feed prescription:
  116.1 g fat daily
  15.3 g protein daily
  23.4 g carbohydrate daily

Recipe
- Use Ketocal as base feed, given in a amount to provide the child's full protein requirements.
- Add additional fat in the form of a long-chain fat module such as Calogen (Nutricia), to meet fat prescription.
- Add additional carbohydrate in the form of glucose polymer such as Maxijul (Nutricia), Vitajoule (Vitaflo) or Caloreen (Nestle) to meet carbohydrate prescription.
- Nutritionally analyse the total mixture to ensure it meets requirements for vitamins, minerals, trace elements and electrolytes.
- If deficient, Phlexy-vit powder (Nutricia) can be added to the feed without altering the carbohydrate content.
- If electrolytes are required and an oral rehydration solution is used to supplement the feed, the additional carbohydrate which it provides must then be deducted from the calculated amount of glucose polymer.

Example recipe
- 100 g Ketocal
- 86 g Calogen
- 21.5 g Maxijul
- Made up to 800 mL with water, provides 1199 kcal (at 1.5 kcal/mL), 15.3 g protein, 116.0 g fat and 23.4 g carbohydrate per total feed.
- This feed provides sufficient vitamins, minerals, trace elements and electrolytes for a boy of 18 months and therefore does not require any further additions.

Table 14.1   Example of phased transition to ketogenic enteral feeds by introducing ketogenic feeds as a percentage of existing enteral feeds.

Phase	Duration	Existing feed	Ketogenic feed
1	1–3 days	75% energy	25% energy
2	1–3 days	50% energy	50% energy
3	1–3 days	25% energy	75% energy
4			100% energy

Table 14.2 Example of phased transition from existing to ketogenic enteral feeds by introducing full ketogenic feeds at a reduced ratio.

Phase	Duration	Ketogenic feed 100% energy
1	1–3 days	2:1
2	1–3 days	2.5:1
3	1–3 days	3:1
4	1–3 days	3.5:1
5		4:1

Box 14.2 Example calculation showing phased transition from normal to ketogenic enteral feed using full ketogenic feed at reduced ratio

- *Aim*: 3:1 ratio, 1200 kcal, 15.3 g protein
- *Initiate at 2:1 ratio*: using dietary unit method (see Chapter 8), total daily enteral feed prescription = 109.1 g fat, 15.3 g protein, 39.25 g carbohydrate, 1200 kcal
  Recipe: 100 g Ketocal, 72 g Calogen, 38 g Maxijul
- *Progress to 2.5:1 ratio*: using dietary unit method, total daily enteral feed prescription = 113.21 g fat, 15.3 g protein, 29.98 g carbohydrate, 1200 kcal
  Recipe: 100 g Ketocal, 80 g Calogen, 28.5 g Maxijul
- *Final recipe for 3:1 ratio feed*: 100 g Ketocal, 86 g Calogen, 21.5 g Maxijul

is shown in Box 14.2, using the figures from the example classical KD enteral feed calculation given in Box 14.1.

Each ratio will require a recalculation; however as the Ketocal quantity is based on the protein requirement, it will remain constant in all ratios, requiring only minor alterations to additional fat and glucose polymer. The initial calculation of a 2:1 ratio feed should highlight any vitamin, mineral, trace element or electrolyte deficiencies; therefore once you have established if the prescribed amount of Ketocal meets nutritional requirements, this will apply for all the other ratio recipes. Repeat analysis should not be needed and further calculations are minor.

Medium-chain triglyceride ketogenic enteral feeds

If a child has a strong history of reflux or has previously not tolerated Ketocal feeds, a modular medium-chain triglyceride (MCT) feed can be used. As with the MCT KD, the MCT enteral feed should induce a greater degree of ketosis allowing a reduction in the total fat required, which may aid tolerance. The MCT modular feed prescription is based on the MCT KD (Box 14.3). This type of feed is usually initiated continuously, progressing to boluses if well tolerated. If a 3-month trial is successful and the modular feed is well tolerated, then it may be worth considering gradually adapting the feed to match the composition of

---

Box 14.3   Constituents of the MCT modular enteral feed prescription

- Long-chain triglyceride (LCT): provides 12–26% of energy, using an LCT module source such as Calogen (Nutricia). Initially all fat should be given as long-chain; this can then be decreased in corresponding amounts as MCT is introduced.
- MCT: provides 45–60% of energy, using an MCT source such as Liquigen (Nutricia). This is increased gradually over approximately 1 week to ensure MCT is tolerated as can cause gastrointestinal side effects if introduced too quickly.
- Protein: provides 10–12% of energy, using a protein source such as Vitapro (Vitaflo) or Protifar (Nutricia).
- Carbohydrate: provides 15–18% of energy, using a glucose polymer source such as Maxijul (Nutricia), Vitajoule (Vitaflo) or Caloreen (Nestle). Less carbohydrate may be necessary to achieve optimal ketosis.
- Vitamins, minerals and trace elements: added to the feed using Paediatric Seravit or Phlexy-vit powder (both Nutricia) as carbohydrate allowance dictates.
- Electrolytes: sodium and potassium chloride added to meet requirements for age.
- Essential fatty acids: walnut oil added as LCT intake is reduced (0.1 mL for every 56 kcal/day).
- Fibre: if usually on fibre feed then Resource Optifibre (Nestle) can be added.

Ketocal to establish tolerance, prior to switching to Ketocal to reduce preparation time and risk of error.

Existing KD therapy patients who subsequently require enteral feeding

There may be certain circumstances in which a child who is already on a KD therapy requires a period of enteral feeding, for example during intercurrent illness or after surgery. In addition, some children who have previously achieved a reasonable oral intake may experience deterioration in their ability to eat sufficient quantities safely and may require top-up enteral feeds or transition to full enteral nutrition to ensure adequate growth. The feed of choice will be largely based on the type of KD therapy the child is currently following.

Classical KD

For short periods of enteral feeding some centres may use Ketocal made up as suggested to 4:1 ratio, or diluted down to 1 kcal/mL with additional water, providing the appropriate volume to meet the child's specific energy requirements. However, if the child is not currently following a ratio of 4:1 it may be advantageous to match actual ratio and calculated requirements rather than forcing a ratio change at a time when other factors may influence outcome. It may be necessary to reduce the diet ratio in certain situations if ketone levels are excessive or if blood glucose is consistently low following illness or surgical intervention. Calculating a feed to meet actual ratio and requirements using Ketocal is shown in Box 14.1.

MCT KD

If a child is currently on an oral MCT KD and needs short-term enteral feeding, the diet prescription can be translated into a modular MCT enteral feed as described above. This will be more complicated to calculate and prepare and may be less well tolerated due to the increase in osmolality caused by adding several different products. The use of the classical KD product Ketocal is therefore recommended as a first choice for all children on an oral MCT KD who require a period of enteral feeding. The transition to Ketocal should be monitored carefully, and may need to be done in a stepwise process, reducing MCT and carbohydrate content gradually.

Modified Atkins diet

If children currently following a modified Atkins diet (MAD) require a period of enteral feeding, it is suggested that they be initiated on Ketocal. This may need modification to a ratio lower than 4 : 1, at least in the introductory stages, to match the carbohydrate content and ketogenic ratio of the MAD.

Reflux

Many children who are enterally fed suffer from reflux and require medical management of symptoms. All current anti-reflux medication should be checked for carbohydrate content and alternative reduced carbohydrate options prescribed where possible.

Children who are having a feed thickener added to their normal feed can continue to use this provided the carbohydrate allowance is not exceeded. Thickeners contain variable amounts of carbohydrate, which will need to be deducted from the carbohydrate allowance of the feed. A useful alternative is Thixo-D Cal Free (Sutherland Health), a thickening agent which is free of calories, carbohydrate, gluten and milk. It is currently not available on routine prescription in the UK, although it can be ordered direct from the manufacturers.

Jejunal feeding

Jejunal feeding should be considered as an alternative feeding route in cases of aspiration risk or severe reflux, retching or vomiting despite optimal medical management. Ketogenic feeds given via nasojejunal or gastrojejunal tube will need to be given continuously as feed will be dispensed directly into the small intestine, bypassing the stomach reservoir. This has considerable social implications for patients and their families. Although feeds administered via nasojejunal or gastrojejunal tube reduce the risk of reflux and aspiration, there is more risk of poor tolerance resulting in abdominal pain or diarrhoea and malabsorption. Feeds may need to be established gradually, increasing the rate and/or ratio as tolerance allows.

Constipation

Constipation can be a considerable problem for enterally fed children. Ketocal multifibre LQ could be used or fibre can be added in suitable quantities, in the form of Resource Optifibre (Nestle). This contains 14 g carbohydrate per 100 g; some centres calculate this carbohydrate into the feed prescription and other centres do not. Children may also require regular laxative medication to ensure normal bowel function.

Weaning off a ketogenic enteral feed

Weaning from a ketogenic enteral feed to an ordinary enteral feed should be approached in the same way as weaning from a KD, following a staged reduction in ratio by reintroducing a percentage of the desired non-ketogenic enteral feed. Those who have had a period of enteral feeding and are returning to oral diet may require a period where enteral feeds and meals are used in combination. For example, if only half of meals are tolerated, then the prescription can be topped up with an enteral feed. To ensure ratio is maintained meals offered during this phase should the 'all-in-one' mixtures. Vanilla Ketocal feeds can be thickened to purée consistency and used orally while establishing oral intake.

References

Hosain, S.A., La Vega-Talbott, M. and Solomon, G.E. (2005) Ketogenic diet in paediatric epilepsy patients with gastrostomy feeding. *Pediatr Neurol* **32**, 81–83.
Kossoff, E.H., McGrogan, J.R. and Freeman, J.M. (2004) Benefits of an all-liquid ketogenic diet. *Epilepsia* **45**, 1163.

Chapter 15

Dietary initiation

Jan Chapple

Yorkhill Children's Hospital, Glasgow, UK

The classical ketogenic diet (KD) initiation practices have their origin in the historical use of periodic fasting to treat epilepsy. This was therefore part of the traditional method of classical KD initiation in countries worldwide, involving admission to hospital for a period of fasting with carbohydrate-free fluids only. Due to the considerable effects of fasting in children and the cost implication of hospital stay, there have been recent studies examining what are safe and effective diet initiation procedures. This chapter discusses protocols for initiating KD therapy and the importance of blood glucose and ketone monitoring during this process.

Initiation protocols

The duration of fast in traditional initiation protocols varied from 12 hours to when the patient achieved adequate ketosis (large ketones), which in practice is often longer than 48 hours, but never exceeded 72 hours in children (Freeman et al., 2007). Serum glucose was monitored. Following initial fast, classical KD meals were usually introduced in one of two ways.

1 One-third of total calorie requirements at desired ratio, increasing daily by a further one-third of total calories, until full calorie requirement is achieved after 3 days, ketogenic ratio remaining constant throughout.
2 Full calorie requirement, initiating at reduced ratio (2 : 1) and increasing the ratio daily until desired ratio is achieved, calories remaining constant throughout.

Many of the studies on the classical KD have used a fasting initiation protocol. Fasting may result in hypoglycaemia, acidosis, nausea, vomiting, dehydration, anorexia, lethargy and a small risk of increase in seizures. Therefore it must only be carried out in hospitalized patients so they can be closely observed and treated as necessary.

Dietary Treatment of Epilepsy: Practical Implementation of Ketogenic Therapy,
First Edition. Edited by Elizabeth Neal.
© 2012 John Wiley & Sons, Ltd. Published 2012 by John Wiley & Sons, Ltd.

There is now retrospective (Wirrell et al., 2002; Kim et al., 2004) and prospective (Bergqvist et al., 2005) evidence indicating that fasting is not necessary to achieve ketosis and that more gradual initiation procedures produce that same seizure control at 3 months with significantly lower frequency and severity of initiation-related side effects, need for medical intervention, and weight loss. However, fasting may lead to a quicker onset of seizure reduction and may still have a role if a more immediate response is desired. Continued use of fasting initiation procedures is therefore based on each centre's individual practice rather than on the basis of efficacy.

Some centres admit children to hospital for classical or medium-chain triglyceride (MCT) KD initiation and education, providing a period of intensive teaching for patients and families and close monitoring during acclimatization to the prescribed diet. This is especially important for infants and younger children. Other centres start KDs at home. Whether initiated as an inpatient or outpatient, both types of KD are built up to a full prescription gradually; protocols for this gradual initiation may vary from centre to centre. An example of two different dietary calculation methods of incremental increase to a full classical KD is shown in Box 15.1. The modified Atkins diet (MAD) and low glycaemic index treatment (LGIT) do not usually involve an initial hospital admission.

A diet should only be started on an outpatient basis if there is good community support from the diet team; this should include daily telephone contact for at least the first week or two. Home and school or nursery visits can be helpful if logistically achievable. Home initiation will reduce stress on children and families as they do not require admission, remaining in their home environment. It also has considerable cost savings. If the diet is started at home, the diet team must be able to provide all education and training in the outpatient setting; this should include the management of possible early side effects such as excess ketosis and hypoglycaemia.

Blood glucose and ketone levels during initiation

Hypoglycaemia is rare, but during dietary initiation there is a particular risk. Blood glucose levels are likely to fall on commencing a low-carbohydrate diet so should be monitored regularly. The frequency of monitoring will decrease as the diet becomes more established. Blood glucose levels should ideally be kept above 3 mmol/L, although many children on KD therapies have a lower blood glucose level than their counterparts on normal diet. This is not problematic unless symptoms develop.

Symptoms of low blood glucose include sweating, pallor, dizziness, becoming cold and clammy, jittery, confused or aggressive. It is generally suggested that hypoglycaemia should be treated when the blood glucose is at or less than 2.5 mmol/L if asymptomatic or if greater than 2.5 mmol/L and symptomatic. Initially, rapidly absorbed carbohydrate should be given, for example two tablespoons of pure fruit

Box 15.1   Example of two calculation methods for classical KD initiation

- Male, aged 7 years, weight 21.15 kg, height 115.3 cm
- Estimated average requirement for energy = 1890 kcal daily (Department of Health, 1991)
- Aiming for 1 g of protein per kg body weight = 21.15 g daily
- Aiming for 3:1 ketogenic ratio = 182.9 g fat, 21.15 g protein and 39.82 g carbohydrate daily

Method A: desired ratio at one-third energy requirements

Day 1
One-third requirements at 3:1 ratio = 630 kcal
60.9 g fat/day = 15.24 g fat per meal × 4 daily
7.05 g protein/day = 1.76 g protein per meal × 4 daily
13.27 g carbohydrate/day = 3.32 g carbohydrate per meal × 4 daily

Day 2
Two-thirds requirements at 3:1 ratio = 1260 kcal
121.94 g fat/day = 30.49 g fat per meal × 4 daily
14.1 g protein/day = 3.53 g protein per meal × 4 daily
26.54 g carbohydrate/day = 6.64 g carbohydrate per meal × 4 daily

Day 3 onwards
Full requirements at 3:1 ratio = 1890 kcal
182.90 g fat/day = 45.73 g fat per meal × 4 daily
21.15 g protein/day = 5.29 g protein per meal × 4 daily
39.82 g carbohydrate/day = 9.96 g carbohydrate per meal × 4 daily

Method B: full requirements, reduced ratio

Day 1
Full requirements at 2:1 ratio = 1890 kcal
171.82 g fat/day = 42.96 g fat per meal × 4 daily
21.15 g protein/day = 5.29 g protein per meal × 4 daily
61.76 g carbohydrate/day = 15.44 g carbohydrate per meal × 4 daily

Day 2
Full requirements at 2.5:1 ratio = 1890 kcal
178.3 g fat/day = 44.58 g fat per meal × 4 daily
21.15 g protein/day = 5.29 g protein per meal × 4 daily
50.17 g carbohydrate/day = 12.54 g carbohydrate per meal × 4 daily

Day 3 onwards
Full requirements at 3:1 ratio = 1890 kcal
182.90 g fat/day = 45.73 g fat per meal × 4 daily
21.15 g protein/day = 5.29 g protein per meal × 4 daily
39.82 g carbohydrate/day = 9.96 g carbohydrate per meal × 4 daily

juice or a sugar-containing (non-diet) carbonated drink (providing approximately 3–5 g carbohydrate). If the symptoms have not improved after 15–20 minutes, this should be repeated. Children over the age of 5 years may require double this amount of carbohydrate to correct hypoglycaemia; older or larger children may require more. Families or carers should also contact the local doctor, as it will be important to monitor blood glucose levels and provide further treatment. If hospital admission is needed, a glucose infusion may be required. Hypoglycaemia should be discussed with local medical teams to establish thresholds for intervention; some centres recommend treatment if blood glucose falls below 3 mmol/L.

Ketone levels can become too high, especially during diet initiation. Symptoms of excess ketosis are rapid panting breathing, increased heart rate, facial flushing, irritability, vomiting and unexpected lethargy. Treatment is as for hypoglycaemia, and again, if the symptoms have not improved after 15–20 minutes, treatment should be repeated and medical advice sought. It may be necessary to alter the diet ratio if ketone levels are persistently excessive. However, increased lethargy and drowsiness are common when starting a dietary treatment, and may just be due to adaptation to the changes in metabolism occurring with the alteration in diet, rather than due to excess ketosis. Levels should be checked prior to intervention.

Children on carbonic anhydrase inhibitor medications, such as topiramate, may be more prone to excess ketosis and have increased risk of metabolic acidosis on commencing KD therapy. Large decreases in bicarbonate levels have been reported in this group (Wilner et al., 1999; Takeota et al., 2002), and close monitoring is needed, especially during diet initiation.

References

Bergqvist, A.G.C., Schall, J.I., Gallagher, P.R., Cnaan, A. and Stallings, V.A. (2005) Fasting versus gradual initiation of the ketogenic diet: a randomised clinical trial of efficacy. *Epilepsia* **46**, 1810–1819.

Department of Health (1991) *Dietary Reference Values for Food Energy and Nutrients for the United Kingdom*. London: HMSO.

Freeman, J.M., Kossoff, E.H., Freeman, J.B. and Kelly, M.T. (2007) *The Ketogenic Diet: A Treatment for Children and Others With Epilepsy*, 4th edn. New York: Demos Medical Publishing.

Kim, D.W., Kang, H.C., Park, J.C. and Kim, H.D. (2004) Benefits of the nonfasting ketogenic diet compared with the initial fasting ketogenic diet. *Pediatrics* **114**, 1627–1630.

Takeoka, M., Riviello, J.J., Pfeifer, H. and Thiele, E.A. (2002) Concomitant treatment with topiramate and the ketogenic diet in pediatric epilepsy. *Epilepsia* **43**, 1072–1075.

Wilner, A., Raymond, K. and Pollard, R. (1999) Topiramate and metabolic acidosis. *Epilepsia* **40**, 792–795.

Wirrell, E.C., Darwish, H.Z., Williams-Dyjur, C., Blackman, M. and Lange, V. (2002) Is a fast necessary when initiating the ketogenic diet? *J Child Neurol* **17**, 179–182.

Chapter 16

Ketone monitoring and management of illness

Hannah Chaffe

UCL-Institute of Child Health and Great Ormond Street Hospital for Children NHS Trust, London, UK

Ketosis is usually monitored at home by parents or carers. Urinary ketones measure acetoacetate and home blood testing measures serum β-hydroxybutyrate (BHB). Levels are initially recorded daily in the morning and evening. Modification of a ketogenic diet (KD) may be required to ensure adequate ketone levels (see Chapter 17). Once a child is established on a diet, monitoring can become less frequent, perhaps once per day or only at times of dietary fine tuning or during illness. On modified KD therapies like the modified Atkins diet (MAD) and low glycaemic index treatment (LGIT), ketones may not always be routinely recorded. This chapter discusses both methods of home ketone monitoring, management of illness and use of appropriate medications.

Measurement of urine ketones

Process

The child passes urine into a receptacle and a urinary dipstick is placed into the urine. The dipstick changes colour, ranging from light pink to mid-pink, to light purple and finally dark purple. The most popular ketone strips read 0, trace, 0.5, 1.5, 4, 8, 16 (mmol/L) and each number correlates with a shade of pink or purple. When the child starts a KD (without fasting) ketone levels will be 0 and usually progress to 8–16 mmol/L (80–160 mg/dL; sometimes referred to as 3+ to 4+) over the next 2 weeks. Although these large ketone levels are aimed for, seizure control is the primary goal and may occur with lower ketones.

Technique for babies and children in nappies

For a morning specimen, put the cotton wool into a clean nappy. The overnight nappy will not be suitable as the urine is contaminated with numerous urinations.

Dietary Treatment of Epilepsy: Practical Implementation of Ketogenic Therapy,
First Edition. Edited by Elizabeth Neal.
© 2012 John Wiley & Sons, Ltd. Published 2012 by John Wiley & Sons, Ltd.

Squeeze the urine from the cotton wool into a receptacle or onto the dipstick. The colour will change and indicate the level of ketosis. For an evening specimen, put on a clean nappy after the bath or evening meal and check the cotton wool before the child goes to sleep.

Reasons for abnormal or inaccurate results

On occasions the urinary dipsticks do not change colour. It is important to ensure that the ketone strips are stored with the lid on. Damp surroundings (like the bathroom) can affect the accuracy of the strips. Measuring urine ketones for a disabled teenager who is menstruating is not recommended, as the urine sample will become contaminated. If the nappy is soiled, the process should be repeated.

Sometimes ketones are very low and this could be due to a number of reasons:

- not enough urine on the dipstick;
- nappy rash cream being applied (some creams and ointments can contaminate the cotton wool);
- the child is developing an illness;
- the child has had some carbohydrate in error;
- the child has been exercising.

Limitations of urine testing

Many children cannot pass urine at set times, so for a family with morning deadlines, urine measurement may not be the most conducive to family life. Some children pass urine very infrequently, so families may wait several hours for a sample to test. This can be frustrating for the families, but is important for the child's safety, particularly in the early days of the diet, or if excess ketosis is suspected.

Measurement of ketones in urine is not as accurate as measurement of blood levels, as a urine level does not indicate the current ketosis, only what has happened in the past few hours. An excess fluid intake can dilute the level of ketosis and dehydration can elevate the level. At present, urinary dipsticks only read up to 16 mmol/L. This has an impact on children who have episodes of excess ketosis, as actual levels cannot be accurately measured.

Blood measurement of ketosis

Home blood ketone monitoring is becoming more popular due to its accuracy and immediacy. It can be done at a set time each day and does not rely upon waiting for a sample to be produced. Instructions are given in Box 16.1. The literature does not suggest that blood ketone recording is being used on a regular basis. However, most of the worldwide centres contributing to the 2009 consensus

Box 16.1   Instructions for using the blood ketone meter

- Wash the child's finger.
- Set the lancet with the needle and have a tissue ready to absorb the excess blood.
- Turn on the blood ketone machine.
- Insert the blood ketone strip and check that it reads KETONE. (It may be necessary to insert the calibration strip each time a new box of ketone strips is used, depending on the machine.)
- Hold the child's fingertip (use the fleshy part to the left or right) onto the end of the lancet machine and press the button (it may be useful to have a person to help distract the child).
- A small drop of blood should appear on the finger.
- Move the machine to the finger and as the strip touches the blood it should be 'collected' by the ketone strip.
- Wait for the machine to start counting down and it should then display the reading.
- If the machine does not start to count down, it could be that there is not enough blood and the process will need to start again with a new ketone strip.
- Record the ketone measurement on the ketone chart.

statement considered that blood ketone recording could be done regularly at home and was a useful clinical tool when urine ketone levels were good but seizures were not controlled (Kossoff et al., 2009).

There is evidence that blood ketone measures may be helpful as a clinical monitoring tool. Van Delft et al. (2010) reported that seizure control correlated better with blood BHB than the daily urine ketone measures. Gilbert et al. (2000) examined serum BHB levels and urine ketones, and reported better seizure control in children on the KD who had higher levels of BHB. However, both these studies involved blood samples analysed in the hospital laboratory rather than at home with hand-held monitors. Many centres that use blood ketone recording recommend that the BHB level should be maintained between 4 and 6 mmol/L, but there is no literature to confirm this at present.

Reasons for abnormal or inaccurate results

Blood ketone machines may become faulty, so it may be helpful to contact the company which made the machine for advice, and to have a supply of blood ketone machine batteries. The child's finger may be contaminated, so it is very important to wash their hands prior to the test.

Limitations of blood testing

The child may dislike having his or her blood ketones recorded as it can be uncomfortable. Some families may find the machine and lancet difficult to work. The testing strips are expensive, so families may find their family doctors reluctant to prescribe them. Many families who use blood ketone testing have only one machine for testing ketones and blood sugars. Most machines are clear about using different strips for each test, but errors can occur.

Management of illness

At times of illness it is important for the family or carers to contact their local family doctor so a child can be assessed, and if they are very worried about the child's health, to attend the local hospital or call an ambulance. It is common for ketone levels to drop just before a child becomes unwell, due to a combination of factors such as the infection itself and decreased physical activity. Changes in medication, especially if steroids are started, can also lower ketone levels. Although ketosis should be maintained during illness if possible, it is more important for the child to get well again. It is also common for seizures to worsen during intercurrent illness so the medical team should always be informed. Emergency treatment can be given as normal. Occasionally ketone levels can become too high during illness, especially if dietary intake is reduced.

If a child is taken to hospital, intravenous dextrose infusions should be avoided and normal saline used. A small amount of glucose may be needed to maintain blood glucose levels if continued intravenous support is necessary. Blood glucose should always be closely monitored, particularly in babies and children under 2 years old.

Vomiting or diarrhoea

The dietary treatment may need to be stopped if a child has diarrhoea and/or vomiting, although milk feeds should not be stopped or diluted in children under 5 years old without first contacting their medical team (NICE, 2009). If the diet is stopped, it is extremely important to still maintain an adequate fluid intake. Drinks should be offered frequently as tolerated; these should be clear, sugar-free liquids like water, sugar-free fizzy drinks and sugar-free squash. If symptoms continue for 24 hours, the child should see the local family doctor, who may prescribe oral rehydration therapy to replenish the body's electrolyte levels. NICE guidelines state that if children under 5 years old have three vomits or six loose stools in 24 hours, they should always see their family doctor, as they are at risk of dehydration (NICE, 2009). If the child is being fed by gastrostomy or nasogastric tube, an appropriate oral rehydration therapy (prescribed by the family doctor) or water (for a limited period) may need to be used in place of feeds to ensure an adequate fluid intake. It is imperative to watch carefully for signs of low blood glucose and/or excess ketosis (see Chapter 15) during this time.

When the child has stopped vomiting, the diet should be reintroduced slowly. If the child is unable to complete meals, the meal constituents should be mixed together so that the food eaten is in the correct ratio of fat to protein and carbohydrate, regardless of the actual amount eaten. If the child is unable to tolerate the full-fat meals due to continued diarrhoea or vomiting, it may be necessary to reduce the fat in the diet for a couple of days by using half the prescribed amount of cream, butter, oil and/or mayonnaise at each meal for a day, and slowly increasing this back to normal over the next couple of days as tolerated. If a child is using Liquigen or MCT oil (both Nutricia) on the MCT KD, the amount may also need to be reduced by half, and then built back up to full strength over 2–3 days. When reintroducing gastrostomy or nasogastric ketogenic feeds, half strength should be initially used for 12–24 hours, then gradually built up to full strength as tolerated over a few days.

The child may need to be given extra calories in the form of extra meals or snacks for a few days after an illness. For example, if the child has been unwell and missed meals for 3 days, one extra meal should be given for three consecutive days when the child is better and tolerating the full diet.

Fever

It is important for the family or carers to contact their family doctor as they would normally if worried about their child's health. An adequate fluid intake should be maintained by offering sugar-free fluids without restriction, and if the child will eat as usual then the diet can be maintained. It may be more acceptable to use a milkshake meal replacement recipe if a child is unable to complete solid meals (see Chapters 8 and 9 for more detail on KD meal replacement recipes).

Nil by mouth guidelines

The literature on KD and general anaesthesia is scarce, with little consensus on management. The most comprehensive study undertaken so far suggests that carbohydrate-free solutions are safe and blood glucose remains stable throughout surgical procedures up to 1.5 hours. The most common effect noted in procedures longer than 3 hours was a significant decrease in pH, requiring intravenous bicarbonate. Current advice therefore suggests monitoring blood pH in procedures over 3 hours and administering intravenous bicarbonate where necessary (Valencia et al., 2002). The KD team should be informed of every child on a KD therapy who is admitted for general anaesthesia or to the paediatric intensive care unit. An individual care plan should be completed detailing the guidelines for management, for example ketone monitoring, blood tests, intravenous fluids, blood sugar and blood gas monitoring.

After surgery, the child's KD therapy should be reintroduced as soon as possible. Some children on a KD may be prescribed a liquid ketogenic meal replacement feed called Ketocal (Nutricia), which can be used as an alternative to solid food when a child is unwell or not able to take their normal KD meals. Ketocal is particularly suitable for enteral feeds, but the amount and dilution needs to be individualized by the dietitian for each child.

Medications

Medications are often unrecognized sources of carbohydrates. If the carbohydrate content of medications and intravenous fluids is not considered, ketosis can be affected and thus seizure control may be compromised (Box 16.2). Prior to diet initiation, all medication such as antiepileptic drugs and antibiotics need to be changed to sugar-free and sorbitol-free alternatives if possible. The pharmacist should be able to advise on the amount of carbohydrate in the medication. Most 'emergency' medications like buccal midazolam and diazepam are suitable for use on the KD. However, some liquid preparations of antiepileptic drugs like clobazam contain varying amounts of carbohydrate. No medication changes should be made during the first 3 months when the diet is being initiated and during fine tuning of the diet if possible.

Many substances ending in '-ose' or '-ol' (apart from cellulose which is suitable) are usually converted to glucose in the body, so are not recommended for the KD (see Chapters 12 and 13). Syrups, elixirs, and chewable tablets usually have higher carbohydrate content than other dosage forms, so it is advisable to avoid these. Some medications may be labelled as sugar-free but have sorbitol added as the sweetener. Although this can be used in the body as carbohydrate, sorbitol-containing products may be preferable to sucrose-containing formulations if no suitable tablet option can be found. Medications containing saccharin are suitable. Suppositories are also suitable. It is possible to measure ketosis to monitor the effect a medication has had on the diet.

Antipyretics and analgesia

There are a number of preparations for lowering a child's temperature and for use during illness or episodes of pain. Sugar-free paracetamol liquid at the correct dose for the child is suitable for use on the KD, for example Medinol. This liquid

---

Box 16.2   Case report illustrating the problem of carbohydrate in medications

Patient S was a 4-year-old boy on the classical KD. His seizures had been much improved on the diet and were now very infrequent. His mother called in some distress to say that his ketones had dropped, seizures had returned, and that he was unwell with a temperature and an ear infection. The KD team reassured her that sometimes illness can cause ketones to drop and seizures to re-occur. She had seen the local family doctor for a prescription of sugar-free antibiotics which she had collected from her local pharmacy. The KD team suggested she check the antibiotic bottle label; on doing so she found that the pharmacist had given her antibiotics with sugar in it. Very upset and cross that she had not checked the bottle, she went back to the doctor for sugar-free antibiotics. Patient S soon recovered from his ear infection and his seizures reduced in frequency again.

preparation can be bought over the counter, is sugar-free and contains no sorbitol. Paracetamol suppositories are also suitable. A variety of ibuprofen preparations are available, for example liquid sugar-free Fenpaed. Nurofen sugar-free liquid contains sorbitol, but Nurofen granules may be suitable for adolescents, older children, and those with a gastrostomy tube. The pharmacist will be able to advise further.

References

Gilbert, D.L., Pyzik, P.L. and Freeman, J.M. (2000) The ketogenic diet: seizure control correlates better with serum beta-hydroxybutyrate than with urine ketone levels. *J Child Neurol* **15**, 787–790.

Kossoff, E.H., Zupec-Kania, B.A., Amark, P.E. et al. (2009) Optimal clinical management of children receiving the ketogenic diet: recommendations of the International Ketogenic Diet Study Group. *Epilepsia* **50**, 304–317.

NICE (2009) *Management of acute diarrhoea and vomiting due to gastroenteritis in children under 5*. National Institute for Health and Clinical Excellence Clinical Guidelines CG84. Available at www.nice.org.uk/CG84.

Valencia, I., Pfeifer, H.H. and Thiele, E.A. (2002) General anaesthesia and the ketogenic diet: clinical experience in nine patients. *Epilepsia* **43**, 525–529.

Van Delft, R., Lambrechts, D., Verschuure, P., Hulsman, J. and Majoie, M. (2010) Blood beta-hydroxybutyrate correlates better with seizure reduction due to ketogenic diet than do ketones in the urine. *Seizure* **19**, 36–39.

Chapter 17

Fine tuning

Gwyneth Magrath

Matthew's Friends Charity and Clinics, Lingfield, UK

A trial period on a diet is recommended before reviewing the benefit of continuing with treatment. This trial is usually for 3 months which allows for the necessary fine tuning required to achieve optimal seizure control. This regimen must allow for the child's growth and well-being along with the control of seizures. After the 3-month trial, if seizure control has improved, the treatment should be continued; ongoing fine tuning of the diet will be necessary to manage treatment and maintain seizure control.

The classical ketogenic diet (KD) is frequently initiated using extra carbohydrate and therefore a lower diet ratio than is likely to be used once the diet is established. In the UK, the modified Atkins diet (MAD) is also frequently started on a more liberal amount of carbohydrate than the recommended 10 g (Kossoff et al., 2006; see also Chapter 10). In both cases the carbohydrate is reduced to establish effective seizure control. The classical KD ratio will be increased by reducing the carbohydrate in this way. In the case of the medium-chain triglyceride (MCT) KD, the percentage of total energy provided from the MCT fat is gradually increased during initiation to ensure tolerance of the MCT and to find the percentage of MCT required for optimal seizure control. A change in blood ketones together with a loss of seizure control at any stage in any of these diet therapies requires dietary review and adjustment. The following should be checked before any dietary changes are made.

- The diet's principles have been understood and are being correctly implemented by the family.
- There have been no dietary indiscretions. These would have to occur on a regular basis to disrupt the ketosis for more than 24 hours.
- There has been no recent illness as this can disrupt both appetite and ketosis.

Dietary Treatment of Epilepsy: Practical Implementation of Ketogenic Therapy,
First Edition. Edited by Elizabeth Neal.
© 2012 John Wiley & Sons, Ltd. Published 2012 by John Wiley & Sons, Ltd.

- There has been no change in medication or brand of medication. All new medication must be checked for carbohydrate and the diet adjusted to accommodate any extra carbohydrate that is contained in these medicines.

A range of fine-tuning options for different KD therapies can then be tried.

Protein manipulation

The amount of protein in the classical and MCT KD is precisely calculated in accordance with patient's age and weight. The low glycaemic index treatment (LGIT) also prescribes protein, although uses household measures rather than exact weights. The protein in these regimens is unlikely to be used as a fine-tuning tool.

The MAD allows generous or free amounts of protein. So when low ketones do not respond to increasing the fat intake and there is accompanying rapid weight gain, over-indulgence in the protein foods may be the cause. The latter are often more palatable than the high-fat foods allowed on the diet (Box 17.1). Offering large portions of protein foods may also mean the full meal cannot be completed. One 8-year old girl within a few days of starting the diet was found to have been offered a fried egg and two rashers of bacon plus fruit and cream for breakfast; she did not complete her meal. A reduction to either an egg or two rashers of bacon enabled the child to finish all her meal. As this was in the initial stages of the diet there was no obvious effect on her level of ketosis.

Conversely, if a patient on the MAD has excessive ketosis and is losing weight, it may be due to a reduced intake of protein as well as fat and carbohydrate (Box 17.2).

Box 17.1   Case report of excessive protein intake on the MAD

Patient L, aged 6 years, was initiated on the MAD with 35 g carbohydrate daily. The carbohydrate was reduced in the first weeks to 11 g daily to improve ketosis. However, the ketone levels remained low but there was some improvement in alertness and interaction. Dietary fat was increased by 15 g per meal daily giving a total of 45 g daily; each dose was given as 30 mL of Calogen (Nutricia) mixed with tea or water flavoured with vanilla essence. The Calogen was introduced gradually, starting with 10 mL per meal daily and increasing to 30 mL per meal daily over 10 days to give a daily total of 90 mL of Calogen or 45 g of fat. There was still only limited improvement in seizure control after 8 weeks. It was then noted she had gained 5 kg (her original weight was normal for her age and height). Further discussions with her family indicated that she had always enjoyed meat and was now eating adult-sized portions. When this was reduced by at least half the amount her ketone levels increased, her seizures improved significantly and her weight stabilized.

Box 17.2   Case report of inadequate protein and fat intake on the MAD

Patient A, aged 12 years, was initiated on the MAD with 35 g carbohydrate daily; this was reduced in the first weeks to 20 g daily. At the initial stage he was slightly overweight. His blood ketone levels were 3–4 mmol/L with occasional hypoglycaemic episodes and his seizure control was significantly improved. However, he lost 7.5 kg within 3 months and a dietary review showed inadequate protein and fat intake. He disliked fat and although he ate more than before, it was insufficient to ensure an adequate energy intake. He ate all his carbohydrate allowance. The first step was to encourage him to eat the high-protein foods allowed on the diet rather than carbohydrate-containing options such as fish fingers, which he preferred but could no longer have. He was willing, for example, to eat low-carbohydrate frankfurter sausages and home-made beef burgers. As he was unable to tolerate further fat as food, fat was given as a drink using Calogen mixed with water and low-carbohydrate flavourings, introduced gradually. He was already quite ketotic and his increased fat intake might have raised his ketosis to an unacceptable level, so his carbohydrate was increased by 1 g per meal and snack to prevent this. This had to be done more than once and a final amount of 33 g of carbohydrate daily was eventually achieved. These changes stabilized his weight loss and maintained his seizure control.

Carbohydrate manipulation

Carbohydrate can be used to adjust ketosis in all KD therapies. Increasing or decreasing carbohydrate in small amounts will change the blood ketones but not significantly change the dietary energy. As carbohydrate is restricted on all the diets, it should be reduced with caution.

Persistent hypoglycaemia or hyperketosis should be treated pragmatically with a dose of carbohydrate but the underlying cause must be found and the diet adjusted accordingly. While this is being done extra carbohydrate top-ups may be necessary, for example 1–2 g carbohydrate given at the meal or snack prior to the time when the ketone levels usually rise or blood glucose falls. As a patient continues successfully on a dietary therapy and seizures reduce, he or she may become more active and this may lead to mild hypoglycaemia and higher than usual ketones. Giving an extra carbohydrate snack before a period of sustained activity (e.g. swimming or dancing) can help by targeting the activity rather than changing the overall diet.

On a well-established classical KD the ketones occasionally become lowered for no apparent reason. If a child's height and weight are as expected, then excess dietary energy is not the cause and it may be necessary to make reductions in the carbohydrate (Box 17.3). This should be done gradually, making only small changes in the amount of carbohydrate at any one time and giving time for a result before making further adjustments. Adapting to the classical KD with its change of food can be difficult for younger patients. They may not complete their meals and then become hyperketotic and nauseous, which compounds the problem (Box 17.4).

Box 17.3   Case report of fine tuning the classical KD by carbohydrate reduction

Patient N, aged 10 years, on the classical KD. Two years after starting the diet he began to have seizures again and his blood ketones were around 3 mmol/L when previously they were 4 mmol/L and above. There was no apparent reason for this drop in levels, but his height and weight were fine so an energy increase had to be avoided. He was finding the diet a problem. With some reluctance, the carbohydrate was reduced by 1 g at each meal, giving a total daily reduction of 4 g, increasing the diet ratio but not significantly decreasing overall energy. This small reduction raised the ketone levels and led to improved seizure control. The change may also have initiated a tightening up of dietary practice which had become relaxed over the 2 years.

Box 17.4   Case report of high ketone levels on the classical KD

Patient J, aged 2 years, began the classical KD on a 2.25 : 1 ratio; he had three meals a day. His seizure control improved immediately. He was difficult to feed from the first and after 3 weeks he had become impossible. His diet ratio had been adjusted to 3.5 : 1 as his initial ketosis was low. He was discovered to have gastro-oesophageal reflux which, although said to be mild, was exacerbated by the high-fat diet resulting in poor intake and vomiting. This meant his full dietary prescription was not being taken resulting in evening blood ketone levels above 5 mmol/L. Anti-reflux medication was prescribed and improved the situation. Carbohydrate top-ups at mealtimes of 1 g were advised and needed to be increased to 2 g while the family worked to establish the diet. The number of meals was also increased to reduce the fat at each mealtime and one of his meals was given as a ketogenic milkshake drink. These measures improved intake and reduced the ketone levels whilst retaining the improved seizure control experienced since the diet began.

The MCT KD carbohydrate allowance is the most liberal of all the diets. When a child needs an increase in ketosis to improve seizure control, reducing the carbohydrate by a small amount will increase the ketone levels. The larger carbohydrate allowance makes this a less onerous option. Conversely, when using the MCT KD and there is ongoing hyperketosis with attendant lethargy and nausea, then an increase in carbohydrate will reduce the ketone levels. These dietary adjustments will make little change to the overall dietary energy.

The initial carbohydrate prescription of the MAD varies between centres (see Chapter 10). This carbohydrate is usually adjusted in the first few weeks of the diet. The more generous carbohydrate prescriptions (those in excess of 10 g daily) are reduced to improve ketosis and seizure control. At this stage if the ketones are still low other measures are required, for example using MCT as described later in this chapter. A patient on the MAD with a poor energy intake and a limited carbohydrate prescription can become overly ketotic. To reverse this, carbohydrate should be increased and food intake encouraged. However, as energy intake improves and the patient adjusts to the diet, the ketone levels may again drop with reduced seizure control. In this instance the carbohydrate will need a gradual reduction (say by 1 g per meal initially) to regain seizure control.

The weight should always be checked at this stage; a large increase may indicate a need to reduce dietary energy, not carbohydrate.

Fat manipulation

Increasing the fat prescription in all KD therapies will potentially increase the patient's ketone levels and seizure control. This change will also increase the dietary energy, which may be a contraindication for use with the obese child or the child of normal weight. Conversely, a reduction in dietary fat can reduce ketosis. This reduction will also reduce the dietary energy and is not a suitable solution for the underweight child.

To increase ketosis on the MCT KD, the amount of potentially more ketotic MCT is increased, with a corresponding reduction in long-chain triglyceride (LCT). This alters the dietary percentages of MCT and LCT but not the total dietary energy or the percentage of energy from protein or carbohydrate. To improve ketone levels and seizure control it is worth trialling a similar exchange of some LCT for MCT in the classical KD and MAD. As with the MCT KD there would be no energy change in the classical KD prescription. It would be expected that the unmeasured LCT allowance of the MAD would naturally reduce as the MCT was introduced into the diet. The exchange of MCT for LCT in this way is useful for a patient who needs to raise ketone levels and is unable to tolerate more fat or reduced carbohydrate in his or her diet (Box 17.5). The MCT should be introduced gradually, as for example in the following.

- Start with 5 mL of Liquigen (Nutricia) per meal (2.5 g MCT).
- Increase Liquigen gradually up to 40 mL per meal or 20 g MCT depending on the child's age and tolerance.
- If more MCT than this is required then a change of diet to the MCT KD should be considered.

Box 17.5   Case report of adding MCT to the MAD to improve efficacy

Patient M, aged 16 years, had seizures successfully controlled with the MAD, but he wished for a trial on a normal diet. This was unsuccessful as his seizures returned while off the MAD. He returned to his previous MAD regimen of 15 g of carbohydrate daily; protein and fat from foods were allowed freely. At each meal 15 g of extra fat was given as 30 mL of Calogen (giving 15 g of LCT per meal, at four meals daily, giving a total of 90 mL of Calogen or 45 g of LCT fat daily). This did not give the expected improvement in seizure control. His urinary ketones remained low. He was of normal weight, so an increase of the dietary fat and therefore an increase of dietary energy was contraindicated. Therefore the 15 g of LCT per meal was exchanged for 15 g of MCT per meal, given as Liquigen. This was done over 10 days, the exchanges being made in small incremental amounts. This gradual introduction of MCT ensured that it was tolerated and that the correct amount required was assessed. This did not change the dietary energy prescribed. Within a week his seizures had improved and he had good levels of urinary ketones.

A child who has routinely high ketones but is otherwise well and gaining height and weight will need no dietary changes. However, if the child appears well but is losing weight it will be necessary to increase the dietary energy. Fat will be an essential part of any energy increase as it is the most concentrated source of calories. Increasing dietary fat may also increase ketosis so must be done in measured increments. It may also be necessary to increase the dietary carbohydrate simultaneously in the same incremental fashion to prevent hyperketosis.

Energy manipulation

Excessive dietary energy on any KD therapy will lead to excessive weight gain which is likely to reduce ketosis. A child whose ketones have gradually become lower needs to have his or her weight checked. On the classical KD or MCT KD, the total energy prescription of the diet can be initially reduced by 50–100 kcal/day, according to age. Further weekly reductions of 50–100 kcal may be necessary until the weight is controlled. This change should improve ketosis and seizure control. A patient on the MAD or LGIT may also need a calorie reduction. Carbohydrate is the only measured nutrient in the MAD; the change therefore is not as straightforward as for other diets. A dietary assessment will be needed to determine the current energy intake and the reduction required to prevent further weight gain. The reduction must be made with several factors in mind. Decreasing the fat alone may reduce the ketosis so the carbohydrate may have to be reduced. This is not advisable if the diet has only 10 g of carbohydrate prescribed daily. It may be the case that the protein intake is excessive and so it alone will need to be reduced (Box 17.1).

On all diets, if there is weight loss even though all the prescribed food is being eaten, an increase in dietary energy is indicated. It is likely in this situation that the current levels of ketosis and seizure control will be good. On the classical and MCT KD start cautiously with 50–100 kcal/day and continue to increase dietary energy in 50–100 kcal increments daily until weight gain is re-established without compromising seizure control. The dietary changes should be made as necessary on a weekly basis. The increased energy prescription will mean that the KDs will have to be recalculated; in some cases it may be best implemented by the introduction of an extra snack. Although the calories will have increased, the classical KD ratio will remain the same and the MCT KD percentage total energy from protein, carbohydrate and fat will remain unchanged.

Weight loss is not uncommon initially on the MAD if advice given on required fat intake is not clear and specific. A full dietary assessment is needed to determine the actual energy intake, what increase is needed for weight gain and whether it is the fat or protein component of the diet that is falling short. It is likely that all the carbohydrate prescription will be eaten and patients may just dislike the extra fat the diet requires. Ketone levels may be raised by increasing the amount of fat to the required level; if necessary extra carbohydrate may be

> **Box 17.6   Case report of initial weight loss in an overweight patient on the MAD**
>
> Patient S, aged 17 years, was obese when she started the MAD. Her diet was initiated on 32.5 g of carbohydrate which was reduced to 26 g within a fortnight as there was only a small improvement in seizure control. Two weeks later her blood ketones rose to 4.5–5 mmol/L and she felt lethargic and unwell. She had lost 6 kg since commencing the diet. The carbohydrate was increased again to 32 g daily to reduce the ketones to an acceptable level for comfort, but not to compromise the weight loss. The increase in dietary energy made by this increase in carbohydrate was only 26 kcal. The weight loss was due to the removal of the high-calorie carbohydrate foods that she had previously enjoyed. The now restricted energy intake contributed to the high ketone levels. As she adapted to the diet, the carbohydrate was reduced over 6 months to 18 g daily and the blood ketones stabilized at 2–3 mmol/L. Her weight was reduced from 101 to 88 kg and she remained well. Her parents wished to continue the diet.

given to control ketone levels. Protein may also need to be increased (Box 17.2); again the amount will be dictated by the shortfall in the current diet and the child's requirements. An initial weight loss on the MAD can be a bonus for overweight patients (Box 17.6), but to ensure that this is both safe and sustained, reviews of diet and weight are essential.

Conclusion

To manipulate these diets to obtain optimal seizure control it is essential that there be ongoing monitoring, which should include growth, levels of ketosis, general health and well-being (see Chapter 18). Knowledge of the dietary intake and compliance with the dietary advice given by the dietitian are also important factors. The fine tuning of all the diets is most successful when the dietitian has a good working relationship with the patient and family. In some cases it may be appropriate to consider switching to a different type of KD therapy (see Chapter 21).

Reference

Kossoff, E.H., McGrogan, J.R., Bluml, R.M., Pillas, D.J., Rubenstein, J.E. and Vining, E.P. (2006) A modified Atkins diet is effective for the treatment of intractable pediatric epilepsy. *Epilepsia* **47**, 421–424.

Chapter 18

Monitoring and side effects

Elizabeth Neal

Matthew's Friends Charity and Clinics, Lingfield, UK

Haematology and biochemistry

Implementation of ketogenic diet (KD) therapy must include regular blood investigations as part of ongoing monitoring. Although each centre will have their own monitoring protocol, most guidelines are similar. A suggestion is summarized in Table 18.1. Some tests are essential, while others can be treated as optional depending on resources. Full blood count should be regularly checked; although rare in clinical practice, there have been reports of haematological disturbances in children following the KD, both impaired neutrophil function (Woody et al., 1989) and alterations in platelet function with an increased tendency to bleeding (Berry-Kravis et al., 2001). Some centres will additionally perform regular clotting screens.

Elevated serum cholesterol and triglyceride levels have been reported in children on the KD (Dekaban, 1966; Chesney et al., 1999; Keene, 2006), although other studies have not found this to be a problem (Schwartz et al., 1989a; Couch et al., 1999). Cardiovascular risk will be more accurately predicted by analysing lipoprotein fractions. Although the KD can significantly increase plasma low-density lipoprotein (LDL) levels and decrease high-density lipoprotein (HDL) levels (Kwiterovich et al., 2003), the full extent of atherosclerotic and inflammatory risk cannot be assessed from such measures alone without further investigation of arterial distensibility. Whereas raised blood lipids are not an immediate indication to stop dietary treatment, they should be closely monitored. Dietary manipulation should be employed wherever possible, aiming to increase polyunsaturated, rather than saturated, fat intakes. In some cases, substitution of long-chain triglyceride (LCT) with medium-chain triglyceride (MCT) sources may be helpful. High cholesterol levels in KD children may trend back towards normal with time on treatment, perhaps due to progressive metabolic adaptation (Groesbeck et al., 2006; Nizamuddin et al.,

Dietary Treatment of Epilepsy: Practical Implementation of Ketogenic Therapy,
First Edition. Edited by Elizabeth Neal.

Table 18.1 Recommendations for blood investigations during monitoring of ketogenic dietary therapy.

Blood investigation	Frequency of monitoring
Essential	
Full blood count including platelets	Baseline, after 3 months, 6 months, then every 6 months
Renal profile (includes sodium, potassium, urea, creatinine, bicarbonate and albumin)	Baseline, after 3 months, 6 months, then every 6 months
Liver profile	Baseline, after 3 months, 6 months, then every 6 months
Calcium, phosphate	Baseline, after 3 months, 6 months, then every 6 months
Magnesium	Baseline, after 3 months, 6 months, then every 6 months
Glucose	Baseline, after 3 months, 6 months, then every 6 months
Cholesterol and triglycerides (the latter preferably fasting*)	Baseline, after 3 months, 6 months, then every 6 months
Free and acylcarnitine profile	Baseline, after 3 months, 6 months, then every 6 months
Vitamins A, D, E	Baseline, after 3 months, 6 months, then every 6 months
Zinc, selenium	Baseline, after 3 months, 6 months, then every 6 months
Recommended	
Blood ketones and free fatty acids	Baseline, after 3 months, 6 months, then every 6 months
Uric acid	Baseline, after 3 months, 6 months, then every 6 months
Further lipid profile: LDL and HDL	Baseline, after 3 months, 6 months, then every 6 months
Optional	
Clotting screen	Baseline, 6 months, then every 12 months
Vitamin C	Baseline, 6 months, then every 12 months
Copper	Baseline, 6 months, then every 12 months
Vitamin B_{12}, folate	Baseline, 6 months, then every 12 months
Ferritin	Baseline, 6 months, then every 12 months

*If the sample is *not* a fasting sample and values are elevated, repeat test on a fasting sample.

2008). The ratio of omega-3 to omega-6 fatty acids within plasma phospholipids will also have an influence on cardiovascular risk; although these will not be measured during routine clinical monitoring, enriching a KD with omega-3 fatty acids may have benefit in ensuring this ratio is kept within normal range (Dahlin et al., 2007).

Nutritional biochemistry should include carnitine (see Chapter 20), zinc, selenium and magnesium. Selenium deficiency has been reported in children on the KD (Bergqvist et al., 2003) and can result in impaired myocardial function (Bank et al., 2008). Hypomagnesaemia has also been reported (Kang et al., 2004); decline in plasma magnesium may be a particular problem in children on the classical KD, despite micronutrient supplementation (Christodoulides et al., 2012). Fat-soluble vitamins should be regularly monitored due to the risk of high levels of vitamins A and E (Christodoulides et al., 2012) and concern about vitamin D status and bone health (see Chapter 19). Although vitamin C is not routinely measured, deficiency has been reported in one KD child who presented with scurvy and oral complications (Willmott and Bryan, 2008).

Haematological and biochemical indices may need to be measured more frequently in some cases if there are particular concerns. Abnormal test results should be repeated, preferably as soon as possible in case there was an error in specimen collection. If a supplement has been prescribed following a low level, repeat tests should be done after 3 months. In some children it will also be necessary to monitor blood levels of certain antiepileptic drugs (AEDs).

Monitoring efficacy

If possible, the patient's seizure frequency should be monitored at home using a diary, including not just numbers, but the different types, and an idea of severity. This will allow assessment of a treatment's efficacy and identification of patterns which will help with dietary fine tuning. A follow-up electroencephalogram (EEG) may be done after several months on a dietary treatment. Other benefits or adverse effects should be recorded, such as any changes in alertness, awareness and responsiveness, sleep patterns, hunger, behaviour and overall quality of life for both the child and the family. At follow-up appointments the neurologist will advise on how to proceed with AEDs; if dietary treatment has been successful it is likely that these can be reduced using a stepwise weaning process.

Growth

Regular monitoring of weight and length or height is essential while on a dietary treatment. There is evidence of impaired growth in children on the KD (Liu et al., 2003; Peterson et al., 2005; Groesbeck et al., 2006); younger children may be more at risk (Vining et al., 2002). Despite the higher protein allowance of the MCT diet, no differences were seen in the growth of children on this diet compared with the lower-protein classical diet (Neal et al., 2008). Long-term follow-up of children treated with the KD in the past suggests that although growth trajectories improve after diet treatment is discontinued, height Z-scores still tend to be low. A survey of 101 patients who had previously been on a KD found 40 % of those who were under 18 years at the time of the survey were still below the 10th percentile height for age (Patel et al., 2010).

The high level of ketones, and frequently acidosis, induced by KD therapy is likely to have an influence on growth, and the option of medication to control acidosis should be discussed if poor growth is a persistent problem. The monitoring of vitamin D levels is essential if growth is poor and if low, supplementary therapeutic doses should be given. Recent evidence points to a fall in insulin-like growth factor (IGF)-1 levels during KD therapy as a likely mechanism for linear growth problems (Spulber et al., 2009).

Children with neurological disability will often have growth measurements that fall well below the expected centiles for age, and this should be taken into consideration when assessing this group. Although standard centile growth charts are generally used, growth charts have been developed specifically for children with cerebral palsy (Day et al., 2007; available to download at www.lifeexpectancy. org/articles); separate charts are included for five different levels of motor impairment. In children who are unable to have standing height or supine length measures, alternative suggested measures are upper arm length, lower leg length or knee height (Stevenson, 1995); tibial length growth curves for cerebral palsy have been published (Oeffinger et al., 2010).

Kidney stones

The reported incidence of kidney stones in children on the KD is higher that of the general paediatric population. Uric acid, calcium oxalate, calcium phosphate or mixed composition stones have been reported in up to 7 % of children on the diet (Hertzberg et al., 1990; Freeman et al., 1998; Furth et al., 2000; Kielb et al., 2000). Risk may be higher with long-term treatment (Groesbeck et al., 2006) and concomitant use of carbonic anhydrase inhibitors such as topiramate or zonisamide (Paul et al., 2010). An increased, or certainly adequate, fluid intake should be maintained in this co-therapy group.

While on KD therapy, urine should be regularly checked for haematuria, including monthly testing at home or by the family doctor. The calcium/creatinine ratio should be checked every 3 months. Monitoring of plasma uric acid will provide an additional indication of risk of developing this type of stone. A renal ultrasound should be done if urine test is positive for blood on three consecutive occasions and is also recommended for children on carbonic anhydrase inhibitor AEDs prior to commencing diet treatment. Routine use of the alkalinizing agent potassium citrate will significantly decrease the prevalence of stones (Sampath et al., 2007; McNally et al., 2009; Paul et al., 2010). Some centres are now prescribing this for all children on KD therapy whereas others may reserve its use for children who have a raised calcium/creatinine ratio.

Gastrointestinal side effects

Gastrointestinal intolerance is a common KD side effect. Vomiting, diarrhoea and abdominal discomfort are frequently reported in studies of the MCT KD (Huttenlocher et al., 1971; Sills et al., 1986; Schwartz et al., 1989b; Mak et al., 1999); this can usually be alleviated by lowering the amount of MCT in the prescription. These problems are not unique to the MCT diet. In a study of 129 children on the classical KD, Kang et al. (2004) reported diarrhoea in 33% and vomiting in 28% of patients during the first 4 weeks of treatment. A systematic review of 27 studies that listed adverse events in a total of 1066 children, mainly on the classical KD, found a lower incidence of gastrointestinal problems: vomiting was reported in 5.5% and diarrhoea in 1.9% (Keene, 2006). In a randomized trial of the classical and MCT KDs, the only statistically significant difference in gastrointestinal tolerability was the higher incidence of vomiting on the classical diet at 12 months, although more children on the MCT diet were reported to have diarrhoea or abdominal pain (Neal et al., 2009) (Table 18.2). These side effects could usually be resolved by dietary manipulation, although this was not the case in five additional children who withdrew from the study within the first 3 months, one with constipation (classical diet), one with vomiting (MCT diet) and three with diarrhoea (MCT diet).

Constipation is frequently reported as a side effect of the KD in clinical practice (Box 18.1), influenced in part by the low fluid intake in many children with associated neurological feeding problems. High-fibre foods should be included in the dietary prescription wherever possible (e.g. curly kale, chinese leaf, rhubarb and spinach) and an adequate fluid intake maintained. It may be necessary to use medications to help relieve constipation. Despite the higher carbohydrate allowance, the purported osmotic effect of MCT, and

Table 18.2 Reported gastrointestinal side effects of the classical and MCT KD at 3 and 12 months.

Side effect	3 months		12 months	
	Classical diet ($N=47$)	MCT diet ($N=42$)	Classical diet ($N=20$)	MCT diet ($N=23$)
Vomiting	13 (28%)	11 (26%)	9 (45%)*	3 (13%)*
Diarrhoea	7 (15%)	6 (14%)	2 (10%)	4 (17%)
Abdominal pain	5 (11%)	8 (19%)	2 (10%)	4 (17%)
Constipation	21 (45%)	14 (33%)	9 (45%)	9 (39%)

*Significant difference between two diets at $P<0.05$.
N, number providing data at that time point.
Source: Neal et al. (2009).

Box 18.1   Case report of child with constipation

Child J was a 5-year-old boy on the MCT KD who was enjoying a variety of meals and taking his MCT as a supplement mixed into food. His mother contacted the dietitian because he had been passing small amounts of watery, offensive-smelling diarrhoea. The dietitian (thinking it was a dietary issue) suggested the MCT supplement was reduced to see if this was causing the diarrhoea, but after a few days this change had not been helpful. She suggested a sample of the watery stool was taken to the local doctor to rule out infection. The nurse had a longer conversation with his mother later on in the week, and it transpired that J had passed only very regular, small amounts of diarrhoea, almost like a leakage. He had not opened his bowels properly for about a week. The nurse suggested that it could be overflow diarrhoea, as he was constipated. She advised mum to see the local doctor, who diagnosed constipation and overflow diarrhoea and prescribed laxatives. He continued on the MCT diet on laxatives. His seizures were much improved, as was his cognitive progress, particularly awareness of his surroundings.

Table 18.3   Side effects of KD treatment.

Side effect	Early/late onset	Reported incidence (%)
Gastrointestinal (vomiting/ nausea, diarrhoea, abdominal pain, constipation)[1,2]	Early and late	1.9–38.7
Raised serum lipids[1,2]	Early and late	2.6–27.1
Increased infections[1,2]	Early and late	0.8–20.9
Hypoglycaemia[1,2]	Early and late	0.8–7.0
Raised serum uric acid[1]	Early and late	1.8–26.4
Renal stones[1,2]	Late	1.3–3.1
Acidosis[2]	Early	0.8–1.9
Dehydration[1,2]	Early	0.3–46.5
Osteopenia and increased fracture risk[1]	Late	14.7
Pancreatitis[1,2]	Early and late	0.1–0.8
Gallstones[2]	Not stated	0.4
Elevated liver enzymes[2]	Not stated	0.2
Protein-losing enteropathy[2]	Not stated	0.2
Lipoid aspiration pneumonia[1,2]	Early and late	0.3–4.7
Cardiomyopathy[1]	Late	0.8
Hypoproteinaemia[1]	Early and late	3.9–5.5
Hypomagnesaemia[1]	Early and late	4.7–10.9
Hepatitis[1,2]	Early and late	2.3–5.4

[1]Kang et al. (2004), prospective study of 129 cases.
[2]Keene (2006), systematic review of 1066 cases.
Source: Cross et al. (2010). Used with permission from BMJ Publishing Group.

the fact that small amounts of MCT are often substituted for LCT in the classical KD to help soften the stools, many children on the MCT KD also have a problem with constipation (Table 18.2) (Neal et al., 2009). Over 25 % of all children in this study needed medication for constipation at some point during their diet treatment.

There is a risk that children with pre-existing gastro-oesophageal reflux will have symptoms exacerbated by a high-fat regimen. Children with this problem should be fully investigated and treated for reflux prior to commencing KD therapy.

Other side effects

The reported incidence of complications attributed to KD therapy is variable (Table 18.3). Other reports include pancreatitis (Stewart et al., 2001; Lyczkowski et al., 2005), basal ganglia injury (Erickson et al., 2003), KD-induced toxicity of the AED sodium valproate (Ballaban-Gil et al., 1998), and cardiac abnormalities including cardiomyopathy and a prolonged QT interval (Best et al., 2000; Bergqvist et al., 2003; Kang et al., 2004; Bank et al., 2008). Additional regular monitoring with echocardiography may be advisable; this will be a clinical decision made on an individual basis.

Conclusion

The most commonly seen side effects of ongoing KD therapy are gastrointestinal (predominantly constipation), hypercholesterolaemia, kidney stones and a slowing of linear growth. Most other complications are rare in clinical practice but do serve as a reminder of the absolute importance of regular review and thorough monitoring. Risk of complications should not preclude use of dietary treatments, but should be taken into account when assessing suitability of any type of diet for a child with intractable seizures.

References

Ballaban-Gil, K., Callahan, C., O'Dell, C., Pappo, M., Moshe, S. and Shinnar, S. (1998) Complications of the ketogenic diet. *Epilepsia* **39**, 744–748.

Bank, I.M., Shemie, S.D., Rosenblatt, B., Bernard, C. and Mackie, A.S. (2008) Sudden cardiac death in association with the ketogenic diet. *Pediatr Neurol* **39**, 429–431.

Bergqvist, A.G., Chee, C.M., Lutcha, L., Rychik, J. and Stallings, V.A. (2003) Selenium deficiency associated with cardiomyopathy: a complication of the ketogenic diet. *Epilepsia* **44**, 618–620.

Berry-Kravis, E., Booth, G., Taylor, A. and Berman, W. (2001) Bruising and the ketogenic diet: evidence for diet-induced changes in platelet function. *Ann Neurol* **49**, 98–103.

Best, T.H., Franz, D.N., Gilbert, D.L., Nelson, D.P. and Epstein, M.R. (2000) Cardiac complications in pediatric patients on the ketogenic diet. *Neurology* **54**, 2328–2330.

Chesney, D., Brouhard, B.H., Wyllie, E. and Powaski, K. (1999) Biochemical abnormalities of the ketogenic diet in Children. *Clin Pediatr* **38**, 107–109.

Christodoulides, S.S., Neal, E.G., Fitzsimmons, G. et al. (2012) The effect of the classical and medium chain triglyceride ketogenic diet on vitamin and mineral levels. *J Hum Nutr Diet* **25**, 16–26.

Couch, S.C., Schwarzman, F., Carroll, J. et al. (1999) Growth and nutritional outcomes of children treated with the ketogenic diet. *J Am Diet Assoc* **99**, 1573–1575.

Cross, J.H., McLellan, A., Neal, E.G., Philip, S., Williams, E. and Williams, R.E. (2010) The ketogenic diet in childhood epilepsy: where are we now? *Arch Dis Child* **95**, 550–553.

Dahlin, M., Hjelte, L., Nilsson, S. and Amark, P. (2007) Plasma phospholipid fatty acids are influenced by a ketogenic diet enriched with n-3 fatty acids in children with epilepsy. *Epilepsy Res* **73**, 199–207.

Day, S.M., Strauss, D.J., Vachon, P.J., Rosenbloom, L., Shavelle, R.M. and Wu, Y.W. (2007) Growth patterns in a population of children and adolescents with cerebral palsy. *Dev Med Child Neurol* **49**, 167–171.

Dekaban, A.S. (1966) Plasma lipids in children treated with the ketogenic diet. *Arch Neurol* **15**, 177–184.

Erickson, J.C., Jabbari, B. and Difazio, M.P. (2003) Basal ganglia injury as a complication of the ketogenic diet. *Mov Disord* **18**, 448–451.

Freeman, J.M., Vining, E.P.G., Pillas, D., Pyzik, P.L., Casey, J.C. and Kelly, M.T. (1998) The efficacy of the ketogenic diet, 1998: a prospective evaluation of intervention in 150 children. *Pediatrics* **102**, 1358–1363.

Furth, S.L., Casey, J.C., Pyzik, P.L. et al. (2000) Risk factors for urolithiasis in children on the ketogenic diet. *Pediatr Nephrol* **15**, 125–128.

Groesbeck, D.K., Bluml, R.M. and Kossoff, E.H. (2006) Long-term use of the ketogenic diet in the treatment of epilepsy. *Dev Med Child Neurol* **48**, 978–981.

Hertzberg, G.Z., Fivush, B.A., Kinsman, S.L. and Gearhart, J.P. (1990) Urolithiasis associated with the ketogenic diet. *J Pediatr* **117**, 743–745.

Huttenlocher, P.R., Wilbourne, A.J. and Sigmore, J.M. (1971). Medium chain triglycerides as a therapy for intractable childhood epilepsy. *Neurology* **1**, 1097–1103.

Kang, H.C., Chung, D.E., Kim, D.W. and Kim, H.D. (2004) Early- and late-onset complications of the ketogenic diet for intractable epilepsy. *Epilepsia* **45**, 1116–1123.

Keene, D.L. (2006) A systematic review of the use of the ketogenic diet in childhood epilepsy. *Pediatr Neurol* **35**, 1–5.

Kielb, S., Koo, H., Bloom, D.A. and Faerber, G.J. (2000) Nephrolithiasis associated with the ketogenic diet. *J Urol* **164**, 464–466.

Kwiterovich, P., Vining, E.P.G., Pyzik, P., Skolasky, M.A. and Freeman, J.M. (2003) Effect of a high fat ketogenic diet on plasma levels of lipids, lipoproteins, and apolipoproteins in children. *JAMA* **290**, 912–919.

Liu, Y.M., Williams, S., Basualdo-Hamond, C., Stephens, D. and Curtis, R. (2003) A prospective study: growth and nutritional status of children treated with the ketogenic diet. *J Am Diet Assoc* **103**, 107–112.

Lyczkowski, D.A., Pfeifer, H.H., Ghosh, S. and Thiele, E.A. (2005) Safety and tolerability of the ketogenic diet in pediatric epilepsy: effects of valproate combination therapy. *Epilepsia* **46**, 1533–1538.

McNally, M.A., Pyzik, P.L., Rubenstein, J.E., Hamdy, R.F. and Kossoff, E.H. (2009) Empiric use of potassium citrate reduces kidney-stone incidence with the ketogenic diet. *Pediatrics* **124**, e300–e304.

Mak, S.C., Chi, C.S. and Wan, C.J. (1999) Clinical experience of ketogenic diet on children with refractory epilepsy. *Acta Paediatr Taiwan* **40**, 97–100.

Neal, E.G., Chaffe, H.M., Edwards, N., Lawson, M., Schwartz, R. and Cross, J.H. (2008) Growth of children on classical and MCT ketogenic diets. *Pediatrics* **122**, e334–e340.

Neal, E.G., Chaffe, H.M., Schwartz, R. et al. (2009) A randomised trial of classical and medium-chain triglyceride ketogenic diets in the treatment of childhood epilepsy. *Epilepsia* **50**, 1109–1117.

Nizamuddin, J., Turner, Z., Rubenstein, J.E., Pyzik, P.L. and Kossoff, E.H. (2008) Management and risk factors for dyslipidemia with the ketogenic diet. *J Child Neurol* **23**, 758–761.

Oeffinger, D., Conaway, M., Stevenson, R., Hall, J., Shapiro, R. and Tylkowski, C. (2010) Tibial length growth curves for ambulatory children and adolescents with cerebral palsy. *Dev Med Child Neurol* **52**, e195–e202.

Patel, A., Pyzik, P.L., Turner, Z., Rubenstein, J.E and Kossoff, E.H. (2010) Long-term outcomes of children treated with the ketogenic diet in the past. *Epilepsia* **51**, 1277–1282.

Paul, E., Conant, K.D., Dunne, I.E. et al. (2010) Urolithiasis on the ketogenic diet with concurrent topiramate or zonisamide therapy. *Epilepsy Res* **90**, 151–156.

Peterson, S.J., Tangey, C.C., Pimentel-Zablah, E.M., Hjelmgren, B., Booth, G. and Berry-Kravis, E. (2005) Changes in growth and seizure reduction in children on the ketogenic diet as a treatment for intractable epilepsy. *J Am Diet Assoc* **105**, 725–726.

Sampath, A., Kossoff, E.H., Furth, S.L., Pyzik, P.L. and Vining, E.P. (2007) Kidney stones and the ketogenic diet: risk factors and prevention. *J Child Neurol* **22**, 375–378.

Schwartz, R.H., Boyes, S. and Aynsley-Green, A. (1989a) Metabolic effects of three ketogenic diets in the treatment of severe epilepsy. *Dev Med Child Neurol* **31**, 152–160.

Schwartz, R.H., Eaton, J., Bower, B.D. and Aynsley-Green, A. (1989b) Ketogenic diets in the treatment of epilepsy: short term clinical effects. *Dev Med Child Neurol* **31**, 145–151.

Sills, M.A., Forsythe, W.I., Haidukewych, D., MacDonald, A. and Robinson, M. (1986) The medium chain triglyceride diet and intractable epilepsy. *Arch Dis Child* **61**, 1168–1172.

Spulber, G., Spulber, S., Hagenas, L., Amark, P. and Dahlin, M. (2009) Growth dependence on insulin-like growth factor-1 during the ketogenic diet. *Epilepsia* **50**, 297–303.

Stevenson, R.D. (1995) Use of segmental measures to estimate stature in children with cerebral palsy. *Arch Pediatr Adolesc Med* **149**, 658–662.

Stewart, W.A., Gordon, K. and Camfield, P. (2001) Acute pancreatitis causing death in a child on the ketogenic diet. *J Child Neurol* **16**, 633–635.

Vining, E.P.G., Pyzik, P., McGrogan, J. et al. (2002) Growth of children on the ketogenic diet. *Dev Med Child Neurol* **44**, 796–802.

Willmott, N.S. and Bryan, R.A. (2008) Case report: scurvy in an epileptic child on a ketogenic diet with oral complications. *Eur Arch Paediatr Dent* **9**, 148–152.

Woody, R.C., Steele, R.W., Knapple, W.L. and Pilkington, N.S. (1989) Impaired neutrophil function in children with seizures treated with the ketogenic diet. *J Pediatr* **115**, 427–430.

Chapter 19

Dietary treatments and bone health

Christina Bergqvist

Children's Hospital of Philadelphia University of Pennsylvania School of Medicine, Philadelphia, USA

Osteoporosis

Epilepsy and osteoporosis are both international health problems with significant morbidity and cost to the individual and society. Osteoporosis is defined as reduced bone mineralization and loss of internal architecture of the bones resulting in fractures (National Institutes of Health, 2000). One in three women and one in five men over the age of 50 will develop osteoporosis and 200 million people worldwide are affected (Sanchez-Riera et al., 2011). Osteoporosis was previously considered a disease of the elderly but is now increasingly diagnosed in children with chronic disorders and even in 'healthy children' (Apkon, 2002; Baroncelli et al., 2005). Between the years 1990 and 2000, there was a 25 % increase in hip fractures worldwide: osteoporosis has become an epidemic (Vestergaard et al., 2005; Johnell and Kanis, 2006).

The cause for this rise is multifactorial and reflects the changes in our fast-paced society over past generations. The composition of our diets has changed: we eat more processed, less nutritious foods (Prynne et al., 2004). Children's consumption of sodas and soft drinks has increased while their use of milk, the only dairy product that is vitamin D fortified in the USA, has decreased (Black et al., 2002). Society as a whole is sedentary, driving instead of walking or biking, and we work longer hours and exercise less. Skin cancer is also increasing, and many choose to 'cover up' during the summer months either with clothes or protective sunscreens. Internal production of vitamin D (which is essential for calcium metabolism) may be minimal in a great portion of the population. Add to this alcohol, tobacco and medication use and our current epidemic of osteoporosis is less surprising (Wosje and Specker, 2000; Black et al., 2002).

Peak bone mass

Peak bone mass (PBM) is the highest bone mass achieved. We acquire 95 % of our bone mass during childhood and as much as 25 % during our adolescent growth spurt. PBM occurs in the late teens in girls and mid-twenties in boys. It is then maintained until the forties, after which a steady decline follows (Janz, 2002). Genetic factors account for 60–80 % of the variability in PBM. If PBM is not reached, osteoporosis and fractures occur. Small changes in PBM can have major effects on the risk of fractures. An increase in PBM by 10 % can reduce the risk of hip fracture by 50 % (Bonjour et al., 2009). Maximizing PBM is a major goal for osteoporosis prevention (Rizzoli et al., 2009).

Epilepsy, fractures and antiepileptic drugs

Epilepsy affects approximately 1 % of the population and more than 50 million people worldwide (Hauser and Nelson, 1989). Seizures are well controlled with medication in the majority, while 30–40 % continue to suffer from seizures with significant morbidity and loss of quality of life (McEwan et al., 2004a). Epilepsy increases the risk for fractures from both falls and medication use (Vestergaard, 2005). Antiepileptic drugs (AEDs) can directly affect bone remodelling or indirectly affect bone health by interfering with vitamin D and calcium metabolism (Fitzpatrick, 2004). There is now an increasing body of evidence suggesting that AED use predisposes the epilepsy patient to poor bone health and that longer duration of treatment and simultaneous use of multiple medications increases this risk (Sheth et al., 2008).

There is more information regarding the osteoporotic effects of older AEDs like phenobarbital, phenytoin, valproic acid and carbamazepine (Sheth et al., 1995; Akin et al., 1998; Kafali et al., 1999; Sato et al., 2001; Boluk et al., 2004). The data on the newer AEDs is sparse and longitudinal studies are generally lacking (Nissen-Meyer et al., 2007; Coppola et al., 2009; Heo et al., 2011). However, newer medications that induce the P450 enzyme systems or cause acidosis could have similar negative effects on bone health.

Nutrition and physical activity

Children with treatment-resistant epilepsy have poor nutritional status in comparison to healthy children. They have a high incidence of comorbidities such as cerebral palsy and mental retardation which contribute to reduced overall activity level and perhaps ability to eat an adequate amount of food, both increasing their risk for poor bone status (Henderson et al., 2002; Volpe et al., 2007). More surprisingly, children with epilepsy but without physical disabilities also have decreased physical activity. Wong and Wirrell (2006) investigated physical activity in 75 children with epilepsy aged 3–17 years and compared them with their siblings. While there was no difference in the younger age groups, the teens with epilepsy participated less in both group and individual sports activities. The numerous benefits of physical activity are well documented and in the epilepsy patient it may also improve self-esteem, social integration and quality of life (McEwan et al., 2004b). Physical activity, strain or loading of the bones is essential for normal bone remodelling and osteoporosis prevention (Janz, 2002).

Ketogenic diet

The ketogenic diet (KD) effectively reduces seizures in children and adults with treatment-resistant epilepsy. There have been no studies measuring falls and injuries but one can assume that by reducing seizures the KD should also reduce falls and injuries. As an important secondary effect, the KD also allows us to reduce the number of AEDs needed to treat the seizures. In several studies of the long-term effects in KD responders treated for at least a year, 20–60 % of children were successfully weaned off all medications and treated with the KD only (Hemingway et al., 2001; Kang et al., 2004; Groesbeck et al., 2006).

Bergqvist et al. (2007) showed that over 50 % of children with intractable epilepsy who were about to start the KD had insufficient vitamin D status (25-OH vitamin D <32 ng/dL), placing them at risk for osteopenia. Supplementation with low-dose vitamin D_3 (400 IU in the multivitamin) while on the KD for the 15 months normalized their vitamin D status. Fewer falls and injuries, reduced number of AEDs, and improved vitamin D status should improve bone status. Despite these bone-preserving changes, osteopenia and fractures have now been reported in several studies of the longer-duration side effects associated with the KD (Hahn et al., 1979; Kang et al., 2004; Groesbeck et al., 2006). Bone changes take time to develop; perhaps not surprisingly, a 7-month short-term study did not find any changes (Bertoli et al., 2002).

Bergqvist et al. (2008) measured bone mineral content (BMC) every 3 months over a 15-month period using dual-energy X-ray absorptiometry (DEXA) in 25 children on the KD. Whole-body and spine BMC for age and height declined by more than –0.5 Z-score per year while height declined –0.5 Z-score per year. These changes occurred in spite of fewer AEDs and improved vitamin D status, suggesting that the bone loss or lack of bone acquisition while on the KD is a vitamin D-independent mechanism. There are likely several mechanisms involved and acidosis may play an important role. Ketone bodies are acidic, yet the pH is usually normal but bicarbonate is low. These changes indicate an insufficient production or increased need for bicarbonate while on the KD. The acid environment may prevent normal BMC accrual and also affect linear growth, which is now documented in several studies (see Chapter 18). Insulin-like growth factor (IGF)-1 is important for bone formation and there is evidence that IGF-1 becomes suppressed during the KD (Laron, 2001; Spulber et al., 2009). It is likely that the failure to accrue BMC while on the KD is multifactorial and may also include disruptions of the growth hormone axis.

Modified diets

There are no publications of bone health in children with epilepsy treated with the newer modified diets, the modified Atkins diet (MAD) or the low glycemic index treatment. There have been studies on low-carbohydrate, high-protein diets used for weight loss in obese adolescents and adults. The results from these studies are mixed, showing increased urinary calcium excretion with a decrease in markers of bone formation, while a 2-year study using DEXA did not find any significant changes in bone mineral density between the two groups (Adam-Perrot et al., 2006; Foster et al., 2010). These populations are very different and there are major differences in the implementation of a low-carbohydrate diet for epilepsy and for weight loss. The obese patient carries extra weight and hence extra strain on the bones, while the epilepsy patient is smaller and less mobile. The calories are restricted for the obese group, while liberalized for the epilepsy patient where our goal is a normal weight gain. The carbohydrate content is reduced to 20 g per day for the first month and then liberalized and more commonly maintained around 40–80 g in the obese patient. The MAD strictly reduces the carbohydrate content to 10 g per day for the first month and then is 'liberalized' to 20 g (Johns Hopkins Hospital protocol; Kossoff and Dorward, 2008). Both diets result in ketoses to a lesser degree than the KD, but should still increase the acid load and could therefore result in osteoporosis. A well-designed, prospective, longitudinal trial of minimally 1-year duration in the epilepsy population will be necessary to answer this question.

Monitoring and treatment(s)

Our goals for using dietary treatments in children with epilepsy are to stop the seizures and to improve quality of life. Improved nutritional status, maximized physical activity and minimized AED exposure can not only prevent osteoporosis but also improve quality of life. When the KD consensus statement was written in 2009, DEXA screening was considered optional by many programmes (Kossoff et al., 2009). However, with this additional information available, yearly monitoring with DEXA is recommended. It is a quick test that takes 30 seconds to 1 minute and can be administered accurately in children. The radiation exposure is minimal, only one-twentieth of a standard chest X-ray. There are published standards for children and Z-score comparisons with age- and sex-adjusted controls should be used (Kalkwarf et al., 2007, 2010; Bianchi et al., 2010; Zemel et al., 2010). All measurements should also be race and height adjusted. Vitamin D should be measured every 6 months while the child is on a dietary treatment. For children with decreasing BMC age- and height-adjusted Z-scores, calcium and vitamin D supplementation should be maximized and exercise strongly encouraged. Children who are not able to ambulate should use a stander to promote weight-bearing to maximize their bone health (Herman et al., 2007).

References

Adam-Perrot, A., Clifton, P. and Brouns, F. (2006) Low-carbohydrate diets: nutritional and physiological aspects. *Obes Rev* **7**, 49–58.

Akin, R., Okutan, V., Sarici, U., Altunbas, A. and Gokcay, E. (1998) Evaluation of bone mineral density in children receiving antiepileptic drugs. *Pediatr Neurol* **19**, 129–131.

Apkon, S.D. (2002) Osteoporosis in children who have disabilities. *Phys Med Rehabil Clin N Am* **13**, 839–855.

Baroncelli, G.I., Bertelloni, S., Sodini, F. and Saggese, G. (2005) Osteoporosis in children and adolescents: etiology and management. *Paediatr Drugs* **7**, 295–323.

Bergqvist, A.G., Schall, J.I. and Stallings, V.A. (2007) Vitamin D status in children with intractable epilepsy, and impact of the ketogenic diet. *Epilepsia* **48**, 66–71.

Bergqvist, A.G., Schall, J.I., Stallings, V.A. and Zemel, B.S. (2008) Progressive bone mineral content loss in children with intractable epilepsy treated with the ketogenic diet. *Am J Clin Nutr* **88**, 1678–1684.

Bertoli, S., Striuli, L., Testolin, G. et al. (2002) Nutritional status and bone mineral mass in children treated with ketogenic diet. *Recenti Progressi in Medicina* **93**, 671–675.

Bianchi, M.L., Baim, S., Bishop, N.J. et al. (2010) Official positions of the International Society for Clinical Densitometry (ISCD) on DXA evaluation in children and adolescents. *Pediatr Nephrol* **25**, 37–47.

Black, R.E., Williams, S.M., Jones, I.E. and Goulding, A. (2002) Children who avoid drinking cow milk have low dietary calcium intakes and poor bone health. *Am J Clin Nutr* **76**, 675–680.

Boluk, A., Guzelipek, M., Savli, H., Temel, I., Ozisik, H. and Kaygusuz, A. (2004) The effect of valproate on bone mineral density in adult epileptic patients. *Pharmacol Res* **50**, 93–97.

Bonjour, J.P., Chevalley, T., Ferrari, S. and Rizzoli, R. (2009) The importance and relevance of peak bone mass in the prevalence of osteoporosis. *Salud Publica Mex* **51** (Suppl. 1), S5–S17.

Coppola, G., Fortunato, D., Auricchio, G. et al. (2009) Bone mineral density in children, adolescents, and young adults with epilepsy. *Epilepsia* **50**, 2140–2146.

Fitzpatrick, L.A. (2004) Pathophysiology of bone loss in patients receiving anticonvulsant therapy. In: Schachter, S.C. (ed.) *Epilepsy and Behavior*. San Diego: Elsevier.

Foster, G.D., Wyatt, H.R., Hill, J.O. et al. (2010) Weight and metabolic outcomes after 2 years on a low-carbohydrate versus low-fat diet: a randomized trial. *Ann Intern Med* **153**, 147–157.

Groesbeck, D.K., Bluml, R.M. and Kossoff, E.H. (2006) Long-term use of the ketogenic diet in the treatment of epilepsy. *Dev Med Child Neurol* **48**, 978–981.

Hahn, T.J., Halstead, L.R. and Devivo, D.C. (1979) Disordered mineral metabolism produced by ketogenic diet therapy. *Calcif Tissue Int* **28**, 17–22.

Hauser, W.A. and Nelson, K.B. (1989) Epidemiology of epilepsy in children. *Cleve Clin J Med* **56** (Suppl Pt 2), S185–S194.

Hemingway, C., Freeman, J.M., Pillas, D.J. and Pyzik, P.L. (2001) The ketogenic diet: a 3- to 6-year follow-up of 150 children enrolled prospectively. *Pediatrics* **108**, 898–905.

Henderson, R.C., Lark, R.K., Gurka, M.J. et al. (2002) Bone density and metabolism in children and adolescents with moderate to severe cerebral palsy. *Pediatrics* **110**, e5.

Heo, K., Rhee, Y., Lee, H.W. et al. (2011) The effect of topiramate monotherapy on bone mineral density and markers of bone and mineral metabolism in premenopausal women with epilepsy. *Epilepsia* **52**, 1884–1889.

Herman, D., May, R., Vogel, L., Johnson, J. and Henderson, R.C. (2007) Quantifying weight-bearing by children with cerebral palsy while in passive standers. *Pediatr Phys Ther* **19**, 283–287.

Janz, K. (2002) Physical activity and bone development during childhood and adolescence. Implications for the prevention of osteoporosis. *Minerva Pediatr* **54**, 93–104.

Johnell, O. and Kanis, J.A. (2006) An estimate of the worldwide prevalence and disability associated with osteoporotic fractures. *Osteoporos Int* **17**, 1726–1733.

Kafali, G., Erselcan, T. and Tanzer, F. (1999) Effect of antiepileptic drugs on bone mineral density in children between ages 6 and 12 years. *Clin Pediatr* **38**, 93–98.

Kalkwarf, H.J., Zemel, B.S., Gilsanz, V. et al. (2007) The bone mineral density in childhood study: bone mineral content and density according to age, sex, and race. *J Clin Endocrinol Metab* **92**, 2087–2099.

Kalkwarf, H.J., Gilsanz, V., Lappe, J.M. et al. (2010) Tracking of bone mass and density during childhood and adolescence. *J Clin Endocrinol Metab* **95**, 1690–1698.

Kang, H.C., Chung, D.E., Kim, D.W. and Kim, H.D. (2004) Early- and late-onset complications of the ketogenic diet for intractable epilepsy. *Epilepsia* **45**, 1116–1123.

Kossoff, E.H. and Dorward, J.L. (2008) The modified Atkins diet. *Epilepsia* **49** (Suppl. 8), 37–41.

Kossoff, E.H., Zupec-Kania, B.A., Amark, P.E. et al. (2009) Optimal clinical management of children receiving the ketogenic diet: recommendations of the International Ketogenic Diet Study Group. *Epilepsia* **50**, 304–317.

Laron, Z. (2001) Insulin-like growth factor 1 (IGF-1): a growth hormone. *Mol Pathol* **54**, 311–316.

McEwan, M.J., Espie, C.A. and Metcalfe, J. (2004a) A systematic review of the contribution of qualitative research to the study of quality of life in children and adolescents with epilepsy. *Seizure* **13**, 3–14.

McEwan, M.J., Espie, C.A., Metcalfe, J., Brodie, M.J. and Wilson, M.T. (2004b) Quality of life and psychosocial development in adolescents with epilepsy: a qualitative investigation using focus group methods. *Seizure* **13**, 15–31.

National Institutes of Health (2000) Osteoporosis prevention, diagnosis, and therapy. *NIH Consensus Statement* **17**, 1–45.

Nissen-Meyer, L.S., Svalheim, S., Tauboll, E. et al. (2007) Levetiracetam, phenytoin, and valproate act differently on rat bone mass, structure, and metabolism. *Epilepsia* **48**, 1850–1860.

Prynne, C.J., Ginty, F., Paul, A.A. et al. (2004) Dietary acid–base balance and intake of bone-related nutrients in Cambridge teenagers. *Eur J Clin Nutr* **58**, 1462–1471.

Rizzoli, R., Bianchi, M.L., Garabedian, M., McKay, H.A. and Moreno, L.A. (2009) Maximizing bone mineral mass gain during growth for the prevention of fractures in the adolescents and the elderly. *Bone* **46**, 294–305.

Sanchez-Riera, L., Wilson, N., Kamalaraj, N. et al. (2011) Osteoporosis and fragility fractures. *Best Pract Res Clin Rheumatol* **24**, 793–810.

Sato, Y., Kondo, I., Ishida, S. et al. (2001) Decreased bone mass and increased bone turnover with valproate therapy in adults with epilepsy. *Neurology* **57**, 445–449.

Sheth, R.D., Wesolowski, C.A., Jacob, J.C. et al. (1995) Effect of carbamazepine and valproate on bone mineral density. *J Pediatr* **127**, 256–262.

Sheth, R.D., Binkley, N. and Hermann, B.P. (2008) Progressive bone deficit in epilepsy. *Neurology* **70**, 170–176.

Spulber, G., Spulber, S., Hagenas, L., Amark, P. and Dahlin, M. (2009) Growth dependence on insulin-like growth factor-1 during the ketogenic diet. *Epilepsia* **50**, 297–303.

Vestergaard, P. (2005) Epilepsy, osteoporosis and fracture risk: a meta-analysis. *Acta Neurol Scand* **112**, 277–286.

Vestergaard, P., Rejnmark, L. and Mosekilde, L. (2005) Osteoporosis is markedly under-diagnosed: a nationwide study from Denmark. *Osteoporos Int* **16**, 134–141.

Volpe, S.L., Schall, J.I., Gallagher, P.R., Stallings, V.A. and Bergqvist, A.G. (2007) Nutrient intake of children with intractable epilepsy compared with healthy children. *J Am Diet Assoc* **107**, 1014–1018.

Wong, J. and Wirrell, E. (2006) Physical activity in children/teens with epilepsy compared with that in their siblings without epilepsy. *Epilepsia* **47**, 631–639.

Wosje, K.S. and Specker, B.L. (2000) Role of calcium in bone health during childhood. *Nutr Rev* **58**, 253–268.

Zemel, B.S., Leonard, M.B., Kelly, A. et al. (2010) Height adjustment in assessing dual energy X-ray absorptiometry measurements of bone mass and density in children. *J Clin Endocrinol Metab* **95**, 1265–1273.

Chapter 20

Carnitine

Elizabeth Neal

Matthew's Friends Charity and Clinics, Lingfield, UK

Background

Carnitine is a small water-soluble compound. It is synthesized in the body, mainly the liver and kidneys, from the amino acids lysine and methionine. Approximately 90% of body stores are in muscle. The term L-carnitine is sometimes used, this isomer being the only biologically active form. Carnitine has an essential role in fat metabolism; long-chain fatty acids must combine with it to form acylcarnitines (esters) in order to be transported into the cell mitochondria for oxidation. This process by which carnitine facilitates the transfer of long-chain fatty acids into the mitochondria is termed the *carnitine shuttle*, as once carnitine has transported the acylcarnitines across the inner mitochondrial membrane it is shuttled back across the membrane for the process to be repeated. Inside the mitochondria oxidation of fatty acids occurs in stages, with two carbons removed at each stage to form acetyl coenzyme A (acetyl-CoA); this either enters the Krebs cycle or is used to synthesize ketone bodies. An important point, explained in more detail later, is that all the intermediates of this oxidation process can combine with carnitine in the mitochondria, forming acylcarnitines. Acetyl-CoA can also combine with carnitine within the mitochondria to form acetylcarnitine; this then leaves the mitochondria with ketone bodies. Medium-chain fatty acids do not require esterification to acylcarnitines; they can pass directly into mitochondria for oxidation. These processes are simplified in Figure 20.1, showing the roles of the enzymes carnitine palmitoyltransferase (CPT)-1, CPT-2 and translocase.

Carnitine is well absorbed from food, the main dietary sources being animal based such as milk, meat and eggs, although endogenous synthesis will normally be adequate to meet the metabolic requirements of adults and children, even if vegetarian.

Dietary Treatment of Epilepsy: Practical Implementation of Ketogenic Therapy,
First Edition. Edited by Elizabeth Neal.
© 2012 John Wiley & Sons, Ltd. Published 2012 by John Wiley & Sons, Ltd.

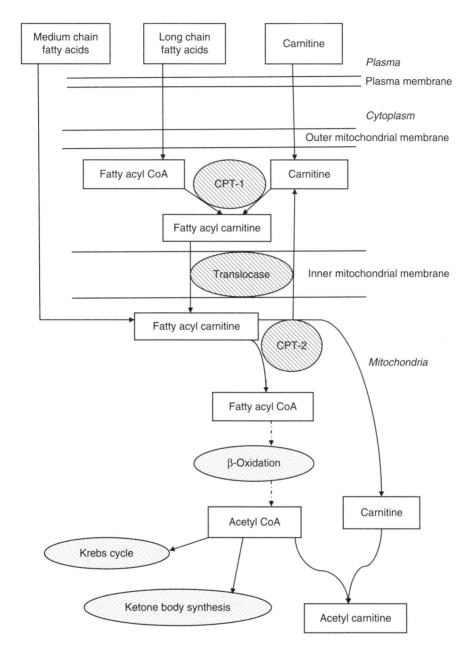

Figure 20.1 Summary of metabolic pathways involved in the carnitine shuttle.

Carnitine and the ketogenic diet

During treatment with a high-fat ketogenic diet (KD) therapy, more carnitine will be needed to facilitate transport of the elevated levels of fatty acids into the mitochondria for oxidation. This will increase risk of depletion of body carnitine stores, a risk that may be further magnified by concurrent food restrictions reducing dietary carnitine intake. There is additional concern for individuals treated with the anticonvulsant medication valproic acid. This has been shown to deplete both muscle and serum carnitine levels in otherwise healthy children with epilepsy (Anil et al., 2009; Hamed and Abdella, 2009), although this has been questioned in other studies (Hirose et al., 1998; Fung et al., 2003): these differences may influenced in part by the health status and therefore dietary intake of the population being studied.

If carnitine status is compromised it will be difficult to achieve adequate ketosis due to impaired ketone body synthesis; energy levels may also be impaired. These concerns are most specifically related to treatment with the classical KD. Because medium-chain triglyceride does not require carnitine for its oxidation process, the modified Atkins diet allows free protein and the low glycaemic index treatment does not actively encourage excess fat intake, these alternative dietary protocols may not pose such a theoretical risk. Scientific data on this subject are limited. There are two studies that address this issue in children on a classical KD.

Berry-Kravis et al. (2001) examined plasma total carnitine levels in 46 patients (age range 1–24 years); this included 38 who were followed from diet initiation, and an additional eight already on the diet at the time of commencing the study. Of the 38 patients monitored from diet initiation, three were started on carnitine supplementation at baseline due to low levels, and five others needed supplementation later in diet treatment (three after 1 month, two after 6 months). One of the additional eight patients already on the diet needed carnitine supplementation due to low levels after 1 year. Therefore, of all the KD patients who were not started on carnitine when starting the diet, six (18 %) went on to have low levels and need supplementation later, none of whom showed any clinical signs of carnitine deficiency or worsening of seizure control. The average total carnitine in patients who were never carnitine supplemented was lower after 1 and 6 months on the diet than at baseline, but this increased again by 12 and 24 months. The conclusion from this study was that total carnitine can decrease over the first few months of KD treatment, and in some patients can dip into the deficiency range, but then normalises with no evidence of a continued decline in levels.

One other study measured plasma free carnitine levels in 164 epilepsy patients (age range 1 month to 6 years), of which 11 were on the classical KD. None of these 11 diet patients developed abnormal levels of free carnitine (Coppola et al., 2006).

Assessing carnitine status and supplementation

The two studies discussed above used total and free carnitine. Total carnitine includes free carnitine and the sum of all the acylcarnitines (carnitine-fatty acid esters), including the intermediates of the fat oxidation process that have combined with carnitine, and acetylcarnitine. In a state of ketosis, even β-hydroxybutyrate will combine with carnitine to form β-hydroxybutyrylcarnitine; these will all be included in the acylcarnitine fraction. Another measure of carnitine status that has been suggested is the ratio of plasma acylcarnitine to free carnitine. A 1998 consensus statement paper on carnitine supplementation in childhood epilepsy (De Vivo et al., 1998) suggested that a free carnitine level of less than 20 μmol/L or a ratio of acylcarnitine to free carnitine greater than 0.4 (after 1 week post term) would indicate a deficiency. These were arbitrary values, and centres may use slightly different age-dependent cut-offs for deficiency. We do not know what measures accurately determine status as plasma levels are not a true reflection of total body stores, most of these being in muscle. Although free carnitine does give a useful indication of status in patients on the KD, the acyl/free ratio does not. Because of the increase in fat metabolism and ketosis that occurs while on the diet, levels of acylcarnitines, including acetylcarnitine, will be greatly increased, and this will result in an elevated ratio. This is a normal consequence of being on the KD, and is likely to reflect the level of ketosis rather than an indication of carnitine status. Indeed, further supplementation with carnitine will have no effect on reducing the ratio, and may even cause it to increase due to increased formation of acetylcarnitine. It has been suggested that the ratio may normalize slightly with time on the KD, due to adaptations to the ketotic state (Berry-Kravis et al., 2001).

There are many anecdotal reports, often from parents or carers, of the benefits of carnitine supplementation (Box 20.1); this can be irrespective of plasma levels. Reported improvements in energy levels can be difficult to assess as the common deficiency symptoms of muscle weakness and tiredness will frequently be present in fluctuating degrees in children with severe epilepsy. Other suggested benefits relate to seizure control, ketone levels, growth and even the reduction of high blood cholesterol levels. A true carnitine deficiency will impair oxidation of fatty acids in the mitochondria and ketone production so a drop in ketone levels would be expected. There are differing views among neurologists with regard to carnitine during KD therapy; some are happy to prescribe it on a trial basis as an additional tool for dietary fine tuning even if levels are normal, while others would look for either biochemical or clinical deficiency before starting treatment. As carnitine can be bought over the counter in health shops, many parents or carers have independently supplemented their KD child, although this is unadvised without informing the KD team.

If carnitine supplementation is used, what is the suggested dose? The 1998 consensus paper recommended supplementing patients with biochemical deficiency at 100 mg/kg body weight daily, in three or four divided doses, up to

Box 20.1   Case report of carnitine supplementation on the classical KD

- Child Y was a boy with Lennox–Gastaut syndrome, diagnosed aged 3 years.
- After trying many anticonvulsant medications without success, he started a classical 4 : 1 ratio KD aged 6 years.
- Seizure control was much improved but he had problems maintaining a stable ketosis and adequate weight gain for growth.
- After 8 months on KD, carnitine supplementation was started and the dose slowly increased to 2 g daily.
- His free carnitine level on KD was low prior to supplementation (12.6 μmol/L compared with 35.9 μmol/L 6 months prior to starting the diet).
- After starting carnitine supplementation both ketone levels and blood glucose stabilized, he started to gain weight, and seizure control improved further, allowing a reduction in anticonvulsant medication.
- Six months after starting carnitine supplementation his carnitine level had improved and he was drug and seizure free.
- Although his seizures did return after a few months following an infection, and the KD was eventually stopped after 2 years of treatment, the family view the time following introduction of carnitine as the most stable period of seizure freedom in the entire history of his epilepsy to date.

a maximum of 2 g/day (De Vivo et al., 1998). The patients studied by Berry-Kravis and her group were given a daily dose of 50 mg/kg of carnitine if deficient. There may be poor absorption, diarrhoea and in some cases even a worsening of seizures if these high doses are started without a gradual build-up. Many centres use a low starting level of 10 mg/kg daily for patients on the KD, which is increased as needed, although individual requirements may differ. Any supplements should contain the L-carnitine isomer only; those also including the D-isomer should be avoided as this may interfere with the absorption and functioning of L-carnitine (Webb, 2006). Absorption of carnitine from supplements may be significantly lower than that from foods (Webb, 2006) so carnitine-rich foods should be included in the diet wherever possible within the constraints of an individual prescription.

Conclusion

The majority of the members of the consensus group on optimal clinical KD management recommended only supplementing carnitine if the patient is biochemically deficient or showing clinical signs of deficiency (Kossoff et al., 2009). However, some parents or carers will want to try carnitine as an option for their child as a fine-tuning tool, even if levels are within normal range. This should always be discussed with the KD team. If supplements are commenced, a low starting dose should be used with a gradual increase and plasma levels should be regularly monitored. Just as with any dietary fine tuning, carnitine should not be added to the prescribed diet at the same time as implementing any other changes so that outcomes can be accurately assessed.

References

Anil, M., Helvaci, M., Ozbal, E., Kalenderer, O., Anil, A.B. and Dilek, M. (2009) Serum and muscle carnitine levels in children receiving sodium valproate. *J Child Neurol* **24**, 80–86.

Berry-Kravis, E., Booth, G., Sanchez, A.C. and Woodbury-Kolb, J. (2001) Carnitine levels and the ketogenic diet. *Epilepsia* **42**, 1445–1451.

Coppola, G., Epifanio, G., Auricchio, G., Federico, R.R., Resicato, G. and Pascotto, A. (2006) Plasma free carnitine in epilepsy children, adolescents and young adults treated with old and new antiepileptic drugs with or without ketogenic diet. *Brain Develop* **28**, 358–365.

De Vivo, D.C., Bohan, T.P., Coulter, D.L. et al. (1998) L-Carnitine supplementation in childhood epilepsy: current perspectives. *Epilepsia* **39**, 1216–1225.

Fung, E.L., Tang, N.L., Ho, C.S., Lam, C.W. and Fok, T.F. (2003) Carnitine level in Chinese epileptic patients taking sodium valproate. *Pediatr Neurol* **28**, 24–27.

Hamed, S.A. and Abdella, M.M. (2009) The risk of asymptomatic hyperammonemia in children with idiopathic epilepsy treated with valproate: relationship to blood carnitine status. *Epilepsy Res* **86**, 32–41.

Hirose, S., Mitsudome, A., Yasumoto, S., Ogawa, A., Muta, Y. and Tomoda, Y. (1998) Valproate therapy does not deplete carnitine levels in otherwise healthy children. *Pediatrics* **101**, e9.

Kossoff, E.H., Zupec-Kania, B.A., Amark, P.E. et al. (2009) Optimal clinical management of children receiving the ketogenic diet: recommendations of the International Ketogenic Diet Study Group. *Epilepsia* **50**, 304–317.

Webb, G.P. (2006) *Dietary Supplements and Functional Foods*. Oxford: Blackwell Publishing.

Chapter 21

Switching or discontinuing dietary treatment

Bridget Lambert

Vitaflo International Ltd, Liverpool, UK

Switching dietary treatment

Neither the classical nor medium-chain triglyceride (MCT) versions of the ketogenic diet (KD) have been found to be significantly better in the management of childhood epilepsy (Neal et al., 2009). The modified Atkins diet (MAD) and low glycaemic index treatment (LGIT) are now widely used and are also proven and effective dietary regimens, particularly for older children, adolescents and adults. It is established that all four types of KD therapy are generally well tolerated and acceptable (Kossoff and Rho, 2009). However, there may be reasons for considering switching to a different version once the child is established or started on a particular diet, including for example the following.

1 Some children, particularly younger ones, may not tolerate all the Liquigen or MCT oil required on the MCT KD due to gastrointestinal side effects. Some may find this and/or the amount of MCT products and food too much to manage comfortably. The classical KD with its smaller meals may suit them better.

2 Some children may prefer the higher carbohydrate intake permitted on the MCT KD to the more restricted intake on the classical KD, MAD and LGIT.

3 Undesirable weight loss or gain may occur on the MAD and LGIT. Energy intake may be better prescribed and hence controlled on the classical or MCT KD.

4 Adolescents may want a more liberalized approach to the diet and prefer the MAD or LGIT to the classical or MCT KD, giving more choice and freedom over what they eat and when.

5 A child may start the classical or MCT KD but it may prove too complicated or onerous for the parents to manage successfully. The family may cope better with the MAD or LGIT, which involve less weighing and measuring.

6 Non-compliance may be improved by trying another version of the diet.

Dietary Treatment of Epilepsy: Practical Implementation of Ketogenic Therapy,
First Edition. Edited by Elizabeth Neal.
© 2012 John Wiley & Sons, Ltd. Published 2012 by John Wiley & Sons, Ltd.

Box 21.1   Switching between dietary treatments

Classical to MCT KD or vice versa
- Calculate diet, meals and snacks.
- Educate parents.
- Swap one meal at a time over a few days or weeks, for example:
  Monday and Tuesday: MCT KD breakfast, classical KD lunch, dinner and snacks
  Wednesday and Thursday: MCT KD breakfast and lunch, classical KD dinner and snacks, etc.

Classical KD to MAD or LGIT
- Educate parents.
- Reduce classical KD to a 1:1 ratio (see advice in section Discontinuing the diet)
- Once this lower ratio is tolerated and with adequate ketone production, start the new regimen.

MAD or LGIT to classical KD
- Calculate diet, meals and snacks.
- Educate parents.
- Increase the ratio of the diet from 1:1 to 2:1, and further if necessary.

MAD or LGIT to MCT KD
- Calculate diet, meals and snacks.
- Educate parents.
- Introduce the MCT source as tolerated, and reduce the amount of long-chain fat at the same time until the desired ratios are attained.
- Decrease the protein and increase carbohydrate in stepwise fashion over a set time period, e.g. a week.

7   Suboptimal ketone production might be enhanced by trying a different version of the diet, for example changing from the MAD, where the ratio is around 1:1, to a classical KD and therefore a higher ratio of 2, 3 or 4:1. Some children may have improved seizure control when changed from the MAD to the 'higher-dose' ketogenic therapy of the classical KD (Kossoff et al., 2010).

Suggestions for ways to change from one diet to another are given in Box 21.1. It is also possible to just be brave and do a straight swap of one diet to another, even in one day! During any dietary changeover ensure the KD team is available to give support. Provide education on any possible complications, for example the potential risk of lower blood glucose or higher ketones if changing over to a diet providing less carbohydrate and more fat.

Discontinuation of dietary treatment

It has been traditionally recommended that a KD therapy be tried for 3 months and if successful (i.e. there is a greater than 50% seizure reduction during this period) to continue it for 2 years (Kossoff et al., 2009). This provides a time frame for parents and children to adhere to the diet and be monitored by the healthcare team. The recommended 2-year period is based on the fact that anticonvulsant drugs are often discontinued at this point in children who become seizure-free. Results from a group of patients with infantile spasms suggest a much shorter duration may have similar outcomes with less risk of growth disturbance (Kang et al., 2011). Conversely, if a diet is efficacious and there are minimal side effects, it can be continued for many years, for example in those who obtain over 90% seizure reduction and children with glucose transporter (GLUT) type 1 deficiency, pyruvate dehydrogenase (PDH) deficiency or tuberous sclerosis complex (Kossoff et al., 2007).

For children who have a positive response to the KD, the prospects for that to continue after a return to a normal diet appear favourable. Martinez et al. (2007) found that of children who became seizure-free on the diet, 80% remained so after it was stopped. Other researchers have reported that being on the diet, even for short periods, has long-term benefits in terms of seizure control and health (Marsh et al., 2006; Patel et al., 2010).

Reasons for coming off dietary treatment, aside from it being a success for 2 years or more, include parents and/or the child wanting to stop, perhaps for social reasons; ineffectiveness (generally after 3–6 months of trying it); concerns over side effects such as poor growth and acidosis; non-compliance; or inadequate ketosis.

At present there is no clear consensus or conclusive research-based evidence on the optimal way to discontinue the KD, or to definitively recommend the time period over which this should occur, although there does not appear to be an increased risk of seizure exacerbation if this is done over weeks rather than months (Worden et al., 2011). However, from review of the available literature and collating the views and experiences of paediatric dietitians regarding their personal practice, the following themes emerge.

- Discontinuation is best done on an individual basis, tailored to patient response. Patient and/or caregiver expectations and what they hope to achieve should be recorded at diet initiation and reviewed at follow-up appointments; these may be helpful in deciding whether to continue or not. The individual risk–benefit of continuation should be evaluated 3 months after starting the diet and then 6 monthly or *at least* annually. The natural history of the seizure disorder should also be considered.
- Withdrawal of an anticonvulsant drug is generally carried out over several weeks or months in a stepwise fashion. A similar pattern and approach is recommended for the discontinuation of a dietary treatment.
- The longer the child has been on the diet, regardless of success, the longer the period of withdrawal advised.
- If the child has become seizure-free or had a greater than 90% seizure reduction, a slow discontinuation is recommended.
- If an adequate level of ketosis was not achieved, it is appropriate for the diet to be stopped more quickly than for a child with high ketones, regardless of the success of the diet.
- Parents can be understandably apprehensive and cautious when their child is coming off a dietary treatment, particularly if it has worked. They often need frequent ongoing support and encouragement during transition to a normal diet.

Concerns regarding the stopping of a dietary treatment

Potentially, withdrawing the diet too quickly may provoke seizures. When the decision is made to discontinue the diet the clinical team responsible for the care of the child must be informed and parents reminded to seek medical advice as appropriate. If seizure activity increases during the weaning-off period it could mean the reduction in fat or increase in carbohydrate is too rapid or the diet more effective than previously thought. Then either the discontinuation should be taken more slowly or a return made to the previous dietary regimen, if it is subsequently decided to remain on the diet.

Whilst each child must be considered as an individual and stopping the diet should be tailored to patient response, doing this in consultation with parents is vital, as from their perspective the process and its speed will depend on many factors. These include anxieties about discontinuing the diet, which if high may mean they may want to do things very slowly; difficulties with compliance necessitating a more rapid return to a normal diet; and how effective they considered the diet had or had not been. It is important to take these and any other concerns into consideration during discussions about discontinuing the diet with parents.

If the diet is successfully stopped but seizures re-occur some time later, parents may wish to start the diet again or opt for medication. For the majority of cases this will be effective (Kossoff et al., 2009).

Planning discontinuation of the diet

Before embarking on the discontinuation of a dietary treatment, calculate the desired energy intake for the child. Use this to determine a 'normal diet', with an appropriate distribution for fat, protein and carbohydrate (e.g. 35 %, 15 % and 50 % of energy, respectively), and hence the amounts of each that you are aiming for. This approach will give structure to your plan (see also Box 21.2). Some

---

Box 21.2 Practical points during discontinuation of a dietary treatment

- Continue blood or urine testing until no ketones have been detected for a few days.
- Continue with seizure monitoring throughout.
- Monitor weight regularly, especially during a lengthy weaning period, to ensure adequate energy intake.
- Continue with micronutrient supplementation until the diet is normalized.
- Advise continued vigilance with regard to food 'extras' being given, for example from peers and well-meaning relatives who are aware the diet is being liberalized.
- The amount of food on the child's plate will alter as the diet is discontinued. This may be disconcerting to parents used to the small KD meals and precise portion control. Provide written guidance, follow-up, reassurance and advice on what a normal healthy balanced diet will look like for the child once off the KD, especially if they have been on it for a long time.

parents will follow the advice they are given to the letter. Others will take matters into their own hands and go at their own speed, especially if they perceive there are no ill effects to normalizing the diet. Some children will find something 'forbidden' or be given food by mistake, meaning the diet ends inadvertently well before it is intended!

Discontinuing the classical KD

The following section gives some guidance and suggestions on discontinuing the classical KD by ratio change or by using foods.

Ratios

- Lower the ratio by 0.25, 0.5 or 1 at a time.
- Make ratio changes every 1–2 weeks, or more slowly, for example every month, depending on the response in terms of seizures and/or ketone levels.
- Alternatively, reduce the ratio meal by meal, snack by snack. For example, for a child on 3:1 ratio diet, start by swapping breakfasts over to a 2:1 ratio, then lunches the following week, etc., until on the new ratio.
- Once ketones disappear, the transition to a normal diet can be made more quickly.
- If parents are familiar with using a computer program for meal and snack calculation, provide them with the amounts of fat, protein and carbohydrate required for each ratio reduction.

Using foods

This approach can be used rather than reducing the ratio and can potentially save time in recalculating recipes, but care should be taken to ensure this is still done in a stepwise fashion. It is best not to change or introduce more than one food item at a time. The following are some suggestions.

- Exchange a proportion of the fat in the diet that is given as cream and/or Calogen (Nutricia) for full cream milk (e.g. 50% of the fat), then after a few days or weeks completely swap over to just using milk.
- Halve the amount of oil or butter and give double the weight of protein or carbohydrate food in the recipe.
- Reduce the amount of fat and increase the amount of protein and carbohydrate one meal at a time. For example, start with breakfasts and change over a period of a week, whilst keeping the rest of the diet ketogenic. Once breakfasts are normal, do lunches. The rest of the diet can be changed in the same way.
- Change snacks to 'normal' foods one at a time over a designated time period, for example a banana rather than a ketogenic cookie.
- Provide parents with written guidance on portion sizes for this approach.

Discontinuing the MCT KD

Discontinuation of the MCT KD should follow a stepwise, gradual process.

- Slowly reduce the amount of MCT and increase the protein and carbohydrate, aiming to ensure total dietary energy is kept as similar as possible.
- This can be achieved by reducing MCT in the diet by 5–10 g increments daily, or possibly per meal and/or snack, depending on the total daily dose. Alongside this reduction, protein can be increased by one exchange daily until normal-size protein portions are achieved; this can then be allowed freely.
- Carbohydrate can then be increased by one carbohydrate exchange daily until normal-size portions are reached then also allowed freely.
- Aim for a normal fat intake as a proportion of daily energy requirements (e.g. 35–40%).
- Additional long-chain fat may need to be added to help meet energy requirements during the transition to a normal diet and whilst the MCT is being reduced. This may be necessary in particular in a diet that had a high percentage of the fat content as MCT.

Discontinuing the MAD and LGIT

As with the classical and MCT KD, discontinuation of the MAD is best done in a stepwise fashion. The amount of fat should be slowly reduced. If using the food choice method, then fat choices can be reduced by one to two choices daily or alternate days. Carbohydrate intake can be increased slowly at the same time, for example by 1 g per meal (i.e. 3–4 g daily) every 3–7 days. Alongside this reduction, protein can be decreased (or increased) until normal-size protein portions are achieved then allowed freely. An alternative way is suggested in the recent update of the KD book written by the ketogenic team at Johns Hopkins Hospital, Baltimore. They recommend discontinuing the MAD by firstly only increasing carbohydrate by 10 g daily every 2 weeks until 60 g/day is reached. At this point, protein sources can be substituted for fat for another 2 weeks; after this, meals should be switched to normal one at a time, adding in one new meal to switch weekly (Kossoff et al., 2011).

Discontinuation of the LGIT is covered in Chapter 11.

For all diet types

The reintroduction of concentrated sources of refined carbohydrates should only take place, and then with caution, once the child is fully established on a normal diet without ill effects. Ketone levels should continue to be monitored until a normal diet is achieved. If at any point there is deterioration in seizure control, then the diet needs to revert to the stage at which this was acceptable.

References

Kang, H.C., Lee, Y.J., Lee, J.S. et al. (2011) Comparison of short- versus long-term ketogenic diet for intractable infantile spasms. *Epilepsia* **52**, 781–787.

Kossoff, E.H. and Rho, J.M. (2009) Ketogenic diets: evidence for short and long-term efficacy. *Neurotherapeutics* **6**, 406–414.

Kossoff, E.H., Turner, Z. and Bergey, G.K. (2007) Home guided use of the ketogenic diet in a patient for more than 20 years. *Pediatr Neurol* **36**, 424–425.

Kossoff, E.H., Zupec-Kania, B.A., Amark, P.E. et al. (2009) Optimal clinical management of children receiving the ketogenic diet: recommendations of the International Ketogenic Diet Study Group. *Epilepsia* **50**, 304–317.

Kossoff, E.H., Dorward, J.L., Miranda, M.J., Wiemer-Kruel, A., Kang, H.C. and Kim, H.D. (2010) Will seizure control improve by switching from the Modified Atkins Diet to the traditional ketogenic diet? *Epilepsia* **51**, 2496–2499.

Kossoff, E.H., Freeman, J.M., Turner, Z. and Rubenstein, J.E. (2011) *Ketogenic Diets: Treatments for Epilepsy and Other Disorders*, 5th edn. New York: Demos Medical Publishing.

Marsh, E.B., Freeman, J.M., Kossoff, E.H. et al. (2006) The outcome of children with intractable seizures: a 3- to 6-year follow-up of 67 children who remained on the ketogenic diet less than one year. *Epilepsia* **47**, 425–430.

Martinez, C.C., Pyzik, P.L. and Kossoff, E.H. (2007) Discontinuing the ketogenic diet in seizure-free children: recurrence and risk factors. *Epilepsia* **48**, 187–190.

Neal, E.G., Chaffe, H.M., Schwartz, R. et al. (2009) A randomised trial of classical and medium-chain triglyceride ketogenic diets in the treatment of childhood epilepsy. *Epilepsia* **50**, 1109–1117.

Patel, A., Pyzik, P.L., Turner, Z., Rubenstein, J. E. and Kossoff, E.H. (2010) Long-term outcomes of children treated with the ketogenic diet in the past. *Epilepsia* **51**, 1277–1282.

Worden, L.T., Turner, Z., Pyzik, P.L., Rubenstein, J.E. and Kossoff, E.H. (2011) Is there an ideal way to discontinue the ketogenic diet? *Epilepsy Res* **95**, 232–236.

Section 3
Broader Applications

Chapter 22

Dietary treatment of epilepsy in infants

Nicole Dos Santos

St George's Hospital, London, UK

Neonates and infants have very specific physiological and nutritional needs. Adequate nutrition is essential for preservation of both physical and mental function. Nutrition plays a key role in the development of multiple organ systems in early life. Early nutrition affects not only brain development, growth and body composition, but also metabolic programming that has possible effects later in life (Tsang et al., 2005). Physiological change in early infancy occurs rapidly, on a daily basis, and adequate nutrition is essential to meet these needs. Infants need to be considered as a separate and individual patient group, with specific nutritional requirements and treatment tailored accordingly.

Use of the ketogenic diet in infants

The ketogenic diet (KD) is now recognized as an accepted treatment for children with intractable epilepsy; however, the only published large randomized controlled trial did not include children between the ages of 0 and 2 years (Neal et al., 2008). There is therefore no first-class evidence for the use of the diet in infancy at present.

Historically, the KD was not recommended for infants, infancy being a critical period for neurodevelopment. Nutritional inadequacies were considered too great, the diet was deemed unpalatable, and there were concerns over immature liver function and lipid metabolism and immature renal systems coping with increased renal loads. In addition, little was known about longer-term adverse effects.

Currently, use of the KD in infants and neonates is still limited, with questions surrounding its safety and efficacy, although interest is increasing. The diet is

Dietary Treatment of Epilepsy: Practical Implementation of Ketogenic Therapy,
First Edition. Edited by Elizabeth Neal.

used as a first-line treatment for glucose transporter type 1 (GLUT1) deficiency syndrome, as well as for pyruvate dehydrogenase (PDH) deficiency (see Chapter 27). Earlier diagnosis is now resulting in more infants starting the KD. Contraindications to the use of the KD, including β-oxidation defects and primary carnitine deficiencies, need to be considered and excluded before starting the diet (Kossoff et al., 2009). If there is any doubt then infants should be started as inpatients, as resulting hypoglycaemia may be life-threatening.

Epilepsies of infancy can be catastrophic, with fewer effective treatments available. There is a critical period where treatment can provide improved outcome. Therefore finding an effective treatment as soon as possible is paramount.

Infantile spasms

Internationally, the KD is increasingly being used to treat infantile spasms (IS) and case–control studies have shown positive results for its use. Also known as West syndrome, IS is a seizure disorder specific to infants. It is associated in many cases with an underlying disorder, or can continue to develop into another type of epilepsy syndrome. There are limited treatment options. These include adrenocorticotropin (ACTH), prednisolone and vigabatrin. All these medications are for short-term use only due to significant and sometimes irreversible side effects. Effectiveness of treatment is usually demonstrated within 2 weeks of treatment onset. Early control of IS (i.e. within 4 weeks of onset) results in better outcomes.

Interest in the use of the KD in IS has resurged recently, particularly in the USA. This is due to a number of reasons: the development of ketogenic feeds that make implementation much easier, increasing expense of medication, and the unlicensing of vigabatrin which has meant that alternative treatments have to be explored. Since 2001, retrospective studies have shown the KD to be effective in infants (Nordli et al., 2001; Eun et al., 2006), including a report of improvements in IS when the diet was used as the initial therapy (Rubenstein et al., 2008). At the Johns Hopkins Hospital, Baltimore, USA, the KD is used widely as first- and second-line treatment for IS (Kossoff et al., 2008). The KD is offered first line if:

- new-onset spasms in young infants (4–5 months old);
- infant is seen within 2 weeks of spasm onset;
- nutrition and health otherwise stable;
- a dietitian is available immediately for an emergency start of the KD;
- the family agrees to ceasing the diet after a 2-week period if shown to be ineffective.

The KD is offered as a second-line treatment in older infants (7–9 months) in whom drug treatments have failed to control their spasms. A prospective study

> **Box 22.1 Case report of failure to thrive in an infant started on the KD (as described in Goyens et al., 2002)**
>
> - A 13-day-old infant presented with seizures, hypotonia and developmental delay. Work-up showed biochemical characteristics of GLUT1 deficiency syndrome and therefore a classical KD was started.
> - The KD provided adequate macronutrient and micronutrient intake with normal to high energy provision of up to 150 kcal/kg per day.
> - Fat contributed to 90% of total energy intake.
> - Over the following 6-week period, the infant lost 10% of pre-diet body weight. Investigations showed low lipase activity in duodenal fluid and changes in the jejunum consistent with symptoms of malnutrition.
> - The diet was altered by replacing 12.5% of LCT with MCT, and provision of pancreatic enzymes.
> - Weight was regained over the following 10 days after amendment of diet.

from the Johns Hopkins Hospital, which enrolled 104 infants between 1996 and 2009, showed that 64% of infants had greater than 50% improvement in spasms after 6 months on KD, while 77% had greater than 50% improvement after 12–24 months (Hong et al., 2010).

In the UK, the KD has been used minimally in IS, mainly due to limited evidence and experience. Additionally, the ongoing ICISS (International Collaborative Infantile Spasms Study), in which drug treatment combinations are being assessed and which is currently enrolling all infants diagnosed with IS, is scheduled to continue until 2014.

The risks associated with using the KD in very young infants are unknown. Goyens et al. (2002) present a case report in which a young infant was started on the diet, but experienced weight loss despite adequate macronutrient and micronutrient provision (Box 22.1). This was corrected on substitution of long-chain triglyceride (LCT) with medium-chain triglyceride (MCT), leading to the suggestions that a formula high in LCT may result in failure to thrive in very young infants. This could be due to a number of factors, such as less efficient fat absorption in neonates and young infants as well as pancreatic insufficiency in neonates exacerbated by secondary protein-energy malnutrition. It is recommended that this should be considered in young infants started on the KD. Adverse effects of the KD were seen in 33% of infants in the Johns Hopkins prospective study. These included constipation, gastro-oesophageal reflux, haematuria, kidney stones, acidosis and hypercalcaemia. Dyslipidaemia was identified in 16% of infants (Hong et al., 2010).

Commercially available formulas for use in the KD

At present, the only formula available commercially in the UK is Ketocal 4:1 (Nutricia). An infant-specific feed has been produced and is in trial phase (Ketocal 3:1) but this is not yet available in the UK. There are some precautions to be considered with regard to the use of these formulas. They do not meet recommended guidelines for nutritional content of infant formulas so are not suitable as a sole source of nutrition without careful consideration of individual nutrients.

Table 22.1 shows a comparison between a regulated standard infant formula, Ketocal 3:1 and Ketocal 4:1. An important consideration is the sodium content of the commercial ketogenic feeds (Ketocal), which are up to double the recommended nutrient intake (RNI) for sodium for infants under 1 year old (1.5 mmol/ kg daily) (Department of Health, 1991). As a comparison, standard infant formula, Ketocal 3:1 and Ketocal 4:1 provide 1.1, 2 and 3 mmol/kg daily respectively at 100 kcal/kg daily (the estimated average requirement for dietary energy for a 3-month-old infant). Because of limited renal concentrating capacity, excretion of excess sodium in infants is inefficient. High intakes of sodium chloride result in increased calcium excretion and increased risk of kidney stone formation. In adult studies, low bone density has been associated with high sodium chloride intakes (Heaney, 1997). The RNI for potassium is also exceeded in the ketogenic feeds. Ketocal 4:1 does not meet calcium requirements and the calcium to phosphate ratio is low.

A further consideration when using commercially available products is that infants feed on demand, with the energy content of formula being the determinant of total volume intake (Cooke et al., 1998). A sufficient protein to energy ratio of the feed is therefore important to ensure the infant is meeting protein requirements.

Caution should be exercised when concentrating feeds and consideration given to the renal solute load in relation to limited urine concentrating capacity in infants.

Implementation of the KD in infants

Feeds should be provided at normal requirements for age. Growth should be monitored, weekly on starting and then fortnightly once established, to ensure centiles are maintained for both weight and length for age. It may be necessary to adapt the dietary prescription frequently during the early months to meet high rates of growth.

Feeding should be on demand unless oral feeds are contraindicated. Gastro-oesophageal reflux can be exacerbated on the diet, and if severe a nasojejunal tube may need to be considered. Severe gastro-oesophageal reflux may also affect the maximum achievable ketogenic ratio. High seizure frequency may also increase risk of aspiration, or increase fatigue and result in insufficient intake. Nasogastric or nasojejunal feeding should also be considered if growth is faltering.

If using a 4:1 ketogenic feed (Ketocal), continuation of breastfeeding or infant formula in combination with this ketogenic feed is the most appropriate method of providing the KD for infants. Implementation is usually started with a 1:1 ratio, increasing to a 3:1 ratio in a stepwise fashion. Some centres in the USA start the diet at a 3:1 ratio, with careful monitoring of blood glucose and ketones. The provision of breast milk or infant formula will help to correct the imbalance of micronutrients in the ketogenic feed. Supplementation of micronutrients may

Table 22.1   Comparison of an example standard infant formula with Ketocal formulations.

Nutrient per 100 kcal	Aptamil 1st	Ketocal 3:1	Ketocal 4:1
Energy (kcal)	100	100	100
Protein (g)	2	2.2	2.1
Carbohydrate (g)	11.1 (lactose)	1 (lactose)	0.4 (glucose syrup)
Fat (g)	5.3 (vegetable oil)	9.7 (palm, soya)	10 (soybean oil)
Vitamin A (µg)	84	75.1	52.1
Vitamin D (µg)	1.8	1.7	0.71
Vitamin E (mg)	1.6	1.1	1
Vitamin C (mg)	14	12	6.2
Thiamin (mg)	0.076	0.1	0.1
Riboflavin (mg)	0.189	0.1	0.1
Folic acid (mg)	18	20	15.1
Vitamin B_6 (mg)	0.06	0.1	0.1
Vitamin B_{12} (µg)	0.27	0.2	0.11
Sodium (mg)	26	45.1	68.5
Potassium (mg)	96	142	110
Chloride (mg)	63	68.8	103
Calcium (mg)	76	120	58.9
Phosphorus (mg)	42	80	58.9
Calcium: phosphorus	1.8:1	1.5:1	1:1
Magnesium (mg)	7.6	15	15.1
Iron (mg)	0.8	1.7	1
Copper (µg)	61	119	82.2
Zinc (mg)	0.76	1.2	0.82
Manganese (mg)	0.011	0.09	0.09
Iodine (µg)	18	22.2	12.3
Selenium (µg)	2.3	3	3

be necessary; if over-provision of nutrients cannot be avoided, it should be checked that these are within safe limits and blood levels should be monitored regularly. If breast milk is expressed, this can be mixed with Ketocal, ensuring each bottle contains the combination feed in the correct ratio. If breastfeeding, a prescribed amount of Ketocal should be given before each breastfeed. This should be based on the theoretical fluid and dietary energy intake for age. This will automatically limit the amount of each breastfeed and provide the correct quantities as per required ratio.

Following UK Department of Health guidelines an infant should be weaned at 6 months of age (Department of Health, 2003) or not before 17 weeks of age (British Dietetic Association, 2010). If there is developmental delay this should be assessed on an individual basis, but weaning should not be delayed longer than necessary to ensure specific windows of opportunity are met. Vitamin drops should be considered for infants who have weaned, as per Department of Health guidelines that if taking less than 500 mL of formula per day then extra vitamins

> **Box 22.2 Meal plan for a 9-month-old infant weighing 8 kg on the classical KD**
>
> - Three meals, two snacks and two milk feeds.
> - Daily requirements would be 800 kcal and approximately 12 g protein.
> - A typical meal would provide 160 kcal, 15.6 g fat, 2.5 g protein and 2.6 g carbohydrate, with snacks and milk feeds equivalent to half a meal.
> - Ketogenic ratio approximately 3 : 1.

A, D and E are required (Department of Health, 1994). Ketovite liquid (Paines & Byrne Limited) is a carbohydrate-free multivitamin supplement that is suitable for use on the KD.

As per weaning guidelines, where infants are weaned on restricted diets, the dietitian should ensure dietary variety with mixed protein sources. The provision of adequate dietary energy to ensure normal growth and development should be a principal determinant of the weaning diet. This should start with purées of fruit and vegetables with added oil, cream and protein powder such as Protifar (Nutricia). Meat and fish can be introduced next; two portions of oily fish per week is recommended for girls and up to four portions per week for boys. Home-made foods are required for weaning as commercial baby foods are too high in carbohydrate, although these can be adapted. An adequate dietary intake of calcium should be ensured, with the ratio of calcium to phosphate being 1.2 to 2 : 1. Foods which are good sources of vitamin C should also be encouraged in the weaning diet, ideally at each meal. Box 22.2 shows an example meal prescription for an infant on the KD.

It is important to progress through weaning stages, increasing textures and variety of foods to ensure appropriate skills are developed and windows of opportunity are met. The introduction of finger foods is an important developmental milestone, with 'bite and dissolve' consistency being the most appropriate for weaning diets. These tend to be high in carbohydrate (e.g. breadsticks, rusks, ricecakes and toast) and will not be appropriate for weaning on the KD. Appropriate finger foods could include boiled carrot sticks, cubes of cheese, avocado, or soft pieces of fruit such as banana, soft pear or slightly cooked apple. Weaning breakfasts on the KD could include slices of omelette or hard-boiled egg, pieces of slightly mashed or soft fruit, with a ketogenic 'yoghurt' made with Ketocal and crème fraiche.

Monitoring the KD in infants

Blood ketones and blood glucose should be checked via a heel prick in the morning and the evening. Urine ketones are not sensitive enough to detect elevated ketones. A low blood glucose of less than 2 mmol/L should be treated by giving a small amount of breast milk or infant formula (30 mL); this should be rechecked after 10–15 minutes. Hyperketosis that is symptomatic should be treated with breast milk or infant formula (30 mL), and blood ketones should be rechecked after 10–15 minutes to ensure these have come down. Persistently raised blood ketones may require fine tuning of the diet, checking weight gain and possibly readjusting calories for growth.

Conclusion

The KD has been shown to be an effective treatment for IS in a recent prospective study, and in a number of smaller retrospective studies. A randomized controlled trial is needed to clarify the role of the KD in IS as compared to medication. The diet remains the primary treatment for infants with GLUT1 deficiency, and is a useful option as a treatment for those with IS and other seizure disorders. It is therefore necessary to continue to develop appropriate resources to meet the needs of these infants and their families. More appropriate ketogenic infant formulas, weaning recipes and support materials (for extended family, nurseries and carers) are needed, as well as the benefit of combined experience in this area as more infants are diagnosed earlier. It is of utmost importance to not ignore developmental progress, as this is easily overlooked when faced with all the other issues. Further research into this emerging area will ensure continued evidence-based use of the KD.

References

British Dietetic Association Specialist Paediatric Group (2010) Position Statement: Weaning infants onto solid foods. Available at www.bda.uk.com/publications/statements/PositionStatementWeaning.pdf

Cooke, R.J., Griffin, I.J., McCormick, K. et al. (1998) Feeding preterm infants after hospital discharge: effect of dietary manipulation on nutrient intake and growth. *Pediatr Res* **43**, 355–360.

Department of Health (1991) *Dietary Reference Values for Food Energy and Nutrients for the United Kingdom*. London: HMSO.

Department of Health (1994) *Weaning and the Weaning Diet*. COMA working group on the weaning diet. London: HMSO.

Department of Health (2003) Infant Feeding Recommendation. Gateway reference 3269. www.dh.gov.uk/en/Publicationsandstatistics/Publications/PublicationsPolicyAndGuidance/DH_4097197

Eun, S.H., Kang, H.C., Kim, D.W. and Kim, H.D. (2006) Ketogenic diet for treatment of infantile spasms. *Brain Dev* **28**, 566–571.

Goyens, P., De Laet, C., Ranguelov, N., Ferreiro, C., Robert, M. and Dan, B. (2002) Pitfalls of ketogenic diet in a neonate. *Pediatrics* **109**, 1185–1186.

Heaney, R.P. (1997) The roles of calcium and vitamin D in skeletal health: an evolutionary perspective. *Food, Nutrition and Agriculture* **20**, 4–12.

Hong, A.M., Hamdy, R.F., Turner, Z. and Kossoff, E.H. (2010) Infantile spasms treated with the ketogenic diet: prospective single-center experience in 104 consecutive infants. *Epilepsia* **51**, 1403–1407.

Kossoff, E.H., Hedderick, E.F., Turner, Z. and Freeman, J.M. (2008) A case-control evaluation of the ketogenic diet versus ACTH for new-onset infantile spasms. *Epilepsia* **49**, 1504–1509.

Kossoff, E.H., Zupec-Kania, B.A., Amark, P.E. et al. (2009) Optimal clinical management of children receiving the ketogenic diet: recommendations of the International Ketogenic Diet Study Group. *Epilepsia* **50**, 304–317.

Neal, E.G., Chaffe, H., Schwartz, R.H. et al. (2008) The ketogenic diet for the treatment of childhood epilepsy: a randomised controlled trial. *Lancet Neurol* **7**, 500–506.

Nordli, D.R. Jr, Kuroda, M.M., Carroll, J. et al. (2001) Experience with the ketogenic diet in infants. *Pediatrics* **108**, 129–133.

Rubenstein, J.E. (2008) Use of the ketogenic diet in neonates and infants. *Epilepsia* **49**, 30–32.

Tsang, R.C., Uauy, R., Koletzko, B. and Zlotkin, S. (2005) *Nutrition of the Preterm Infant*, 2nd edn. Cincinnati, OH: Digital Educational Publishing Ltd.

Chapter 23

Dietary treatment of epilepsy in adults

Susan Wood

Matthew's Friends Charity and Clinics, Lingfield, UK

The evidence

The use of ketogenic diet (KD) therapy in the management of epilepsy in adults predates the widespread use of anticonvulsant medications. In 1930, the first study of 100 adults on KD treatment as monotherapy for epilepsy was published (Barborka, 1930). Despite positive results indicating that 12 became seizure-free and a further 44 showed definite benefit (56% achieved a greater than 50% reduction in seizures), it was a further 69 years before the next adult trial was published with similar findings. In this trial a KD was used in addition to antiepileptic drugs (AEDs) in 11 adults (Sirven et al., 1999). Since then, five more adult studies have been published, with variable results, indicating a growing interest in exploring dietary therapy as an option for patients with refractory epilepsy (Table 23.1). No randomized controlled trial has been conducted and total patient numbers included in these prospective studies have been small.

Additional benefits

For many adult patients seeking dietary therapy, it is not simply seizure frequency or the uncertainty of when the next seizure will strike, but also the epilepsy-related problems that impact on the quality of life between seizures, that make life a challenge. Often in difficult cases, many AEDs are used in combination to reduce seizure frequency but this requires a careful balance between maximizing seizure control on the one hand while minimizing drug toxicity on the other. Quality of life may be significantly impaired by drug effects such as cognitive impairment, sedation and metabolic bone disease (Cascino, 2008). Patients also

Table 23.1   Prospective studies on KD therapy in adults.

Reference	Number of patients	Age range (years)	Dietary treatment	Number of patients achieving ≥50% seizure reduction
Kossoff et al. (2008)	30	18–53	Modified Atkins diet	10 (33%)
Carrette et al. (2008)	8	31–55	Modified Atkins diet	1 (13%)
Mosek et al. (2009)	9	23–36	Classical ketogenic diet	2 (22%)
Klein et al. (2010)	12	24–65	Classical ketogenic diet	6 (50%)
Smith et al. (2011)	18	18–55	Modified Atkins diet	3 (17%)

report problems controlling body weight and depression. It is for these subjective aspects relating to the quality of life that diet therapy has the potential to offer a unique range of benefits to adults. Many of the studies have referred to these anecdotal benefits: 'mental conception is clearer' (Barborka, 1930); 'improved thinking and mood without any reduction in AEDs' and 'one patient continued the diet because of improvement in cognition' (Sirven et al., 1999); 'mood improved in all patients completing the study' (Carrette et al., 2008); and 'the changes in the quality of life were unrelated to the accompanying changes in the frequency of the seizures' (Mosek et al., 2009). In addition, weight loss is commonly reported as a side effect of the diet therapy (Carrette et al., 2008; Kossoff et al., 2008; Mosek et al., 2009; Klein et al., 2010; Smith et al., 2011), making it particularly beneficial for those patients who are overweight or obese at the start. Steady weight gain alongside a reduction in seizure frequency has also been shown to be possible if required (Smith et al., 2011).

Increasing demand for treatment

The psychosocial and financial costs of epilepsy are immense and in the UK resources of the National Health Service are finite. Therefore, finding ways in which patients can be empowered to take on an element of personal responsibility for the management of their long-term medical condition would appear both logical and attractive to all concerned. KD therapy would seem to fit this ethos perfectly. However, in 2011, there are fewer than 20 adults on supervised KD therapy in the UK and many of these have struggled to gain medical support. This is because most adult neurologists (and adult dietitians) are unfamiliar with the metabolic theories underpinning dietary therapy for epilepsy or the practicalities of modern-day practice. It is rarely presented as an option on the treatment 'menu' for adults with intractable epilepsy and readily dismissed as being 'too complex', 'unhealthy', 'having many side effects' and 'of no benefit in adults'.

However, dietary therapy is not necessarily a treatment choice for all. Two adult studies reported that only 14 % (Smith et al., 2011) and 34 % (Klein et al., 2010) of medically screened and eligible patients with refractory epilepsy opted to participate in the dietary trials. The remainder declined for reasons such as reluctance to give up their regular diet, the complexity of the diet and cost, despite knowing that no other optional treatment was available (Klein et al., 2010).

Who should be considered for adult KD therapy?

Indications and contraindications for considering KD therapy are essentially the same as for children (Box 23.1). However, adults are free to make their own choices and must be willing and able to take full control of their dietary treatment. Adult patients generally have an immense struggle obtaining supervised diet therapy and therefore most of the patients currently under treatment are self-selected. The following should be considered.

Box 23.1   Indications and contraindications for dietary treatment in adults

Indications
- Epilepsy difficult to control with AEDs
- Side effects from AEDs significantly affecting quality of life
- Late diagnosed metabolic disorders: glucose transporter type 1 (GLUT1) deficiency and pyruvate dehydrogenase (PDH) deficiency

Contraindications (or caution should be exercised)
- Fatty acid oxidation defects
- Organic acidurias
- Familial hyperlipidaemia
- Diabetes mellitus (medication adjustment/monitoring required)
- Hypertension (medication adjustment/monitoring required)
- Gastro-oesophageal reflux (manage prior to referral)
- Dysphagia (manage prior to referral)
- Eating disorders (medically diagnosed) or patients with significant self-imposed food restrictions (manage prior to referral)
- Multiple food allergies

Note: If the patient has a history of bowel problems or irritable bowel symptoms it may be worth screening them for coeliac disease as KD therapy is by nature practically gluten-free and symptomatic improvement could occur by default. For details of the neurological manifestations of gluten sensitivity (including epilepsy) refer to Hadjivassiliou et al. (2010)

Ability to cope with the daily practicalities of shopping, cooking and monitoring

Epilepsy can start at any age. Some adult patients may have had a normal healthy childhood and a fully independent adult life before developing medically intractable epilepsy. Others may have had disabling epilepsy since childhood and not had the opportunity to trial KD therapy while under paediatric care. Consequently, the range of social circumstances, levels of independence and food-related support vary immensely and must be given careful consideration early on in discussions about KD therapy. The following are key areas that need to be explored in adult patients.

- Are they single, living independently and capable of managing alone?
- Are they supported, perhaps still living with parents or have a supportive partner?
- Do they 'eat out' frequently due to work-related travel or perhaps attend day care or respite care facilities?
- Are they living in a community care facility where there may be many carers involved in shopping and food provision?
- Are there any food preferences or religious dietary laws or social aspects of eating that would make it more difficult for them to adjust their diet?
- Do they have a restricted income or claim state benefits?
- Are they able to monitor their therapy by keeping food records, seizure diaries, testing ketone levels and checking their weight regularly?

Some difficulties may only become apparent during the pre-trial assessment period.

Patient/carer expectations of diet therapy

The majority of adult patients referred for (or seeking) KD therapy will have been prescribed a large number of AEDs in varying combinations over many years. In some cases vagal nerve stimulation or surgery will also have failed, so their expectations of diet therapy are generally modest. However, the use of a validated quality-of-life assessment tool may be helpful as a basis for discussions at this stage so that the expectations of patients and/ or carers can be realistically matched (or not) to the potential benefits reported when the therapy is successful. The possibility of side effects should always be discussed.

KD therapy should be considered as would an additional AED, with (ideally) any non-diet treatment changes occurring prior to a 3-month trial period. If the patient is responsive, it may be possible to start to taper AED dosage after 3 months but this cannot be guaranteed.

Implementation of adult KD therapy

Adult protocol is generally 'borrowed' from paediatric practice as there is little practical experience with adults to inform otherwise. Ideally the management team should include a dietitian, neurologist and epilepsy nurse specialist. Support from a pharmacist on medication changes to lower carbohydrate intake can be invaluable in complex cases. Pre-diet medical investigations (Box 23.2) and nutritional assessment (Box 23.3) are essential.

Which dietary treatment?

Adult case experience in the UK is limited but evolving slowly via a cautious experimental approach. Treatments are based on UK paediatric protocols, internationally published papers and the practical experience of dietetic colleagues treating adults in the USA and South Africa. Although adults can use any of the different types of KD therapy, most adult treatments are a hybrid, starting out with one particular regimen such as the modified Atkins diet (MAD) (Box 23.4), but readily incorporating beneficial elements of another. This 'modified ketogenic therapy' could include a MAD-based regimen with

---

Box 23.2   Medical investigations required before KD therapy

- *Renal ultrasound*: for those with a family history of renal calculi or on topiramate, zonisamide or acetazolamide.
- *Biochemical assessments*: as for paediatric treatments, it is important that adults are monitored at baseline and throughout the course of their treatment (see Chapter 18). Any significant deficiencies or abnormalities should be dealt with prior to starting diet therapy.
- *Bone density (DEXA) scan*: this is recommended in view of the potential adverse effects of AED treatment on bone mineralization and vitamin D metabolism (see Chapter 19).

Box 23.3   Assessment of current diet and nutritional status

Diet history
- Discussion of current dietary intake and eating patterns
- Analysis of three (or more) days of typical food intake
- Food preferences and restrictions
- Food allergies and intolerances
- Feeding or swallowing difficulties and any texture modification required
- Fluid intake and types of fluid favoured
- Any behavioural issues with food

Anthropometric assessment
- Height, weight and body mass index (BMI) at baseline
- Discussion of weight history and feelings about weight loss, weight gain or maintenance of current weight

Box 23.4   Case report of the benefit of the MAD diet

- A 44-year-old male who experienced first seizure at age 34 and was diagnosed with temporal lobe epilepsy.
- Treatment with a range of AEDs over the years had some impact on seizure frequency but quality of life was severely impaired by fatigue, loss of mental clarity, chronic gastrointestinal problems (mainly diarrhoea) and recurrent viral infections.
- At age 41, weaned off AEDs and gained an improvement in symptoms, but seizures increased from six to twelve per month.
- After 7 months off AEDs, commenced a 20-g carbohydrate daily MAD regimen and within 3 months seizures reduced to fewer than one per month.
- Now into fourth year on dietary treatment as monotherapy.
- His main difficulties have been practical: living alone and needing to do all his own shopping and cooking. Food intolerances have further limited his diet, making it difficult for him to eat out.

Box 23.5   Case report of the use of a 'modified ketogenic therapy' dietary treatment

- A 27-year-old female with severe refractory epilepsy and a history of recurrent status epilepticus.
- Epilepsy diagnosed at 1 year and well controlled until aged 14 then worsened.
- Trialled KD age 14 and despite evidence of seizure reduction, found classical KD regimen too hard to follow.
- At age 25, started dietary treatment again but this time using a 50-g carbohydrate daily regimen based on the MAD, with added MCT.
- After 2 months she achieved a significant improvement in seizure severity and frequency; also became notably more alert.
- Now she is approaching 2 years on dietary treatment with the main side effect being difficulty maintaining weight, although this has been achieved with dietary manipulation.

additional medium-chain triglyceride (MCT) to enhance ketosis and allow more carbohydrate to be taken (Box 23.5), or the use of low glycaemic index treatment (LGIT) in preparation for a more rigorous carbohydrate-controlled MAD regimen. In some cases, a general carbohydrate restriction without following a particular prescribed diet protocol will produce benefits. Hence there may be some value in a standardized stepwise approach so that the minimal level of intervention is trialled before moving on to the next level (Figure 23.1). Until we have robust clinical evidence to guide us otherwise, the choice of regimen depends on the clinical needs, the social needs and the wishes of the individual.

Enteral feeding

As with the paediatric patient (see Chapter 14), an enteral feed for an adult on KD therapy will be generally based on a classical KD regimen. Depending on body weight and the protein and energy requirements of the adult, a 3 : 1 ketogenic ratio may be more practically achieved than a 4 : 1 ratio. As there are

Basic low glycaemic index (GI) approach and regular moderate meals

There is anecdotal evidence from a few UK adults that there may be changes in seizure pattern and an improvement in overall quality of life as a result of a simple reduction in carbohydrate (CHO)/calorie intake

Key advice points

- Plan regular moderate meals with one to three small snacks
- Focus on switching high GI CHO sources for lower GI CHO sources at **most** meals. Provide a list of low/medium and high GI CHO sources and offer lower GI ideas for breakfast as this is often the meal given the least time and effort yet requiring the most significant adjustment
- Make moderate reductions to CHO portion sizes
- If weight loss is not desired, advise using full fat dairy products and more generous servings of vegetable oils in cooking/salad dressings, etc.
- Ensure adequate fluid intake,from sugar-free sources
- Advise vitamin/mineral supplementation where biochemically indicated or where dietary analysis indicates a poor range of food sources and potential deficiency

Step one

Based on modified Atkins diet (MAD)

Key advice points

- Daily CHO intake is restricted to 15–20 g, independent of calorie requirement
- CHO exchanges are used as a means to control intake and allow variety of fruits and vegetables. CHO is generally distributed evenly through the day
- Encourage generous portions of fats/oils/ high fat foods and provide guidance on portion sizes and distribution, particularly if weight loss is a concern
- Balance meals with a source of protein, a source of fat and a source of CHO
- Ensure adequate fluid intake, from sugar-free sources
- Full spectrum vitamin/mineral supplement normally recommended
- Provide menu guidance based on individual food preferences and lifestyle

Low glycaemic index treatment (LGIT)

Key advice points

- Daily CHO intake is restricted to approximately 10% of energy intake
- Only foods with a GI value of less than 50 are included
- Low GI CHO exchange lists are used
- Encourage generous portions of fats/ oils/high-fat foods sand provide guidance on portion sizes and distribution, particularly if weight loss is a concern
- Ensure adequate fluid intake, from sugar-free sources
- Full spectrum vitamin/mineral supplement normally recommended
- Provide menu guidance based on individual food preferences and lifestyle

Step two

The classical or MCT ketogenic diet may be the regime of choice for some

- Depending on the body weight and the protein and energy requirement of the adult, a classical 3:1 ketogenic ratio may be more practically achieved than a 4:1 ratio

Figure 23.1 A suggested stepwise approach to adult dietary treatment options.

no commercially available ketogenic formulas for adults, feed options tend to be based on one of the following.

1   Modular components: protein, fat (long chain and MCT) and carbohydrate sources with the addition of electrolytes, vitamins and minerals.
2   Ketocal (Nutricia) with additional protein, carbohydrate, vitamins and minerals as required.
3   Pulmocare (Abbott): a reduced carbohydrate feed with energy provided as 27% carbohydrate, 56% fat and 17% protein. This can be very useful as a 'step-down' feed, particularly in cases where tolerance of a high-fat intake may be questioned.

Barriers to use of dietary treatment in adults

No randomized controlled trials have been conducted

All adult KD evidence is from prospective studies. Hence, national guidance in the UK (NICE, 2004) states that 'The ketogenic diet should not be recommended for adults with epilepsy'. This guidance is currently under review and will likely carry no positive or negative recommendation but simply suggest the need for a better class of research evidence. There is an urgent need for a randomized controlled trial to measure the impact of KD therapy on seizure rates, quality of life, and economic variables in adults.

Concerns about the safety of high-fat diets in adults

The high-fat element of these diets causes considerable concern to adult health-care professionals and patients alike. Most adult studies report an increase in total cholesterol fractions and KD treatment protocols ensure that the lipid profile is measured at baseline and then every 3–6 months onwards. If required, steps can be taken to influence lipid fractions by altering dietary fat sources, but each case should be assessed individually. There has been some interesting work published on the potential value of low-carbohydrate regimens in the management of obesity, type 2 diabetes and metabolic syndrome, in terms of weight loss, increased serum high-density lipoprotein cholesterol, increased low-density lipoprotein particle size, reduced serum triglyceride levels and improved sensitivity to insulin (Nordmann et al., 2006; Shai et al., 2008; Volek et al., 2009). Therefore it is possible that the flat glucose/insulin profiles and the significant metabolic shift from fat storage towards fat oxidation induced by the KD may convey additional metabolic benefits to some adults with refractory epilepsy.

A lack of KD knowledge and experience in the adult epilepsy world (neurologists, dietitians and patients)

Amongst the adult epilepsy population with refractory epilepsy there is little awareness that modifications to food choice can have an impact on seizure frequency and associated symptoms. Those adults wishing to trial KD therapy have immense problems obtaining clinical support. At present the lack of funded dietetic time and clinicians with experience of adult KD therapy are significant barriers.

Future directions

The therapeutic benefits of KD therapies are not simply limited to the management of seizures. There is considerable research interest in their impact on a range of intractable neurological conditions affecting adults, such as Parkinson's disease, Alzheimer's disease and some types of brain cancer (see Chapter 28). Future years could see use of KD therapies in adults expand rapidly as the research evidence base grows, both including and beyond epilepsy to these wider potential applications.

References

Barborka, C.J. (1930) Epilepsy in adults: results of treatment by ketogenic diet in one hundred cases. *Arch Neurol Psychiatry* **23**, 904–914.

Carrette, E., Vonck, K., De Herdt, V. et al. (2008) A pilot trial with modified Atkins' diet in adult patients with refractory epilepsy. *Clin Neurol Neurosurg* **110**, 797–803.

Cascino, G.D. (2008) When drugs and surgery don't work. *Epilepsia* **49**, 79–84.

Hadjivassiliou, M., Sanders, D.S., Grunewald, R.A., Woodroofe, N., Boscolo, S. and Aeschlimann, D. (2010) Gluten sensitivity: from gut to brain. *Lancet Neurol* **9**, 318–330.

Klein, P., Janousek, J., Barber, A. and Weissberger, R. (2010) Ketogenic diet treatment in adults with refractory epilepsy. *Epilepsy Behav* **19**, 575–579.

Kossoff, E.H., Rowley, H., Sinha, S.R. and Vining, E.P. (2008) A prospective study of the modified Atkins diet for intractable epilepsy in adults. *Epilepsia* **49**, 316–319.

Mosek, A., Natour, H., Neufeld, M.Y., Shiff, Y. and Vaisman, N. (2009) Ketogenic diet treatment in adults with refractory epilepsy: a prospective pilot study. *Seizure* **18**, 30–33.

NICE (2004) *The Epilepsies: The diagnosis and management of the epilepsies in adults and children in primary and secondary care*. National Institute for Health and Clinical Excellence. Available at www.nice.org.uk/nicemedia/pdf/CG020NICEguideline.pdf

Nordmann, A.J., Nordmann, A., Briel, M. et al. (2006) Effects of low carbohydrate vs low fat diets on weight loss and cardiovascular risk factors: a meta-analysis of randomised controlled trials. *Arch Intern Med* **166**, 285–293.

Shai, I., Schwarzfuchs, D., Henkin, Y. et al. (2008) Weight loss with a low carbohydrate, Mediterranean, or low fat diet. *N Engl J Med* **359**, 229–241.

Sirven, J., Whedon, B., Caplan, D. et al. (1999) The ketogenic diet for intractable epilepsy in adults: preliminary results. *Epilepsia* **40**, 1721–1726.

Smith, M., Politzer, N., MacGarvie, D., McAndrews, M.P. and Del Campo, M. (2011) Efficacy and tolerability of the modified Atkins diet in adults with pharmacoresistant epilepsy: a prospective observational study. *Epilepsia* **52**, 775–780.

Volek, J., Fernandez, M.L., Feinman, R.D. and Phinney, S.D. (2009) Carbohydrate restriction has a more favourable impact on the metabolic syndrome than a low fat diet. *Lipids* **44**, 297–309.

Chapter 24

Ketogenic dietary therapy in India

Janak Nathan

Shushrusha Hospital, Mumbai, India

Introduction to use of the ketogenic diet in India

Use of the ketogenic diet (KD) was started in India in 1996 by Dr J. Nathan after training at the Johns Hopkins Hospital, Baltimore, USA with Dr J. Freeman and Ms Millicent Kelly. The first problem was the difficulty in using American recipes in India. To 'Indianize' the recipes, a team of dietitians led by the author actually prepared Indian recipes using different caloric and ketogenic ratio values. These were carefully weighed, prepared and tasted by the team. Slowly, a bank of 100 recipes was fashioned and a book prepared with basic instructions included. However, as India is multilingual we had to translate these into at least three Indian languages. A few of our patients were so illiterate that they could not read Roman numerals and therefore this had to be taught before they could use the weighing scale.

There was however a lot of negative feedback from other physicians initially. In fact, one family physician persuaded the parents to stop the diet after one child developed an incidental urinary tract infection, convincing the family that the ketones in the urine were the cause. Luckily the child's infantile spasms had already stopped and there were no more seizures after just 4 months on the diet. There was also a lot of resistance to the use of fasting in the initial phase of introduction of the KD. This was more from the parents than the children, who went through this phase without much fuss. However, we soon realized that hospitalization also entailed a fair expense to the parents, especially as most Indians do not have medical insurance. So, in late 1997 a short carbohydrate washout period was introduced during which very low to zero carbohydrates were given. As there was no fasting phase, we stopped hospitalization, thus reducing the initiation to 2 days. Patients reached urine ketone levels of 4+

Dietary Treatment of Epilepsy: Practical Implementation of Ketogenic Therapy,
First Edition. Edited by Elizabeth Neal.

(160 mg/dL, 16 mmol/L) in 2–4 days and the calculated KD was started after this. Since 1998 we have been using a total outpatient approach.

We have begun using lower ketogenic ratios for the classical KD and have been able to show that lower ratios are as effective as higher ratios as long as good urine ketone levels of 4+ are maintained. Therefore, in our centre we begin with a lower ratio (2 to 2.5 : 1) and if the urine ketone levels are not sufficiently high (i.e. less than 4+) then we increase the ratio or calories. If the ketones are too high we reduce the ratio. Of 79 patients specifically evaluated for lower and higher ratios, 15 patients were on high ratio, i.e. above 3 : 1 (six between 3.1 and 3.5 : 1 and nine above 3.5 : 1) and 49 were on lower ratios, i.e. below 3 : 1 (one between 1 and 1.5 : 1, six between 1.6 and 2 : 1, 22 between 2.1 and 2.5 : 1 and 20 between 2.6 and 3 : 1). Seizure reduction was not significantly different in the two groups (low ratio and high ratio): 51.3 % of patients had 90–100 % seizure reduction in the low ratio group while 65.7 % of patients had 90–100 % reduction in the high ratio group. In both groups, 34.3 % of patients had 50–90 % reduction.

In our centre we also offer KD therapy to adults. Since 1996 we have treated 21 adults, 20 adolescents, 92 children and eight infants with the KD in our centre. Responder rate (>50 % control) has been 81.8 % for infants, 80 % for children, 100 % for adolescents and 42.9 % for adults. Over 90 % reduction in seizures was seen in 45.4 % of infants, 45.5 % of children, 33.3 % of adolescents and 28.6 % of adults.

India has a large number of vegetarians, including some who will not eat anything that grows below the ground, for example onions, potatoes and garlic. Also, culinary practice varies every 100–200 km. Therefore, recipes have to be tailor-made depending on the region of origin.

Use of soy

The protein content of vegetarian food is low and therefore we started using soy as a source of vegetable protein. The advantages are many. Compared with a Western KD, where protein is mainly of animal source, in the Indian KD protein is largely from soybean products. Soy is associated with a decrease in the risk of coronary heart disease. Naturally occurring isoflavones in soy reduce the plasma concentrations of total and low-density lipoprotein (LDL) cholesterol (Potter et al., 1998). Soybean is a rich source of the phospholipid lecithin. Lecithin has been used as a treatment for high cholesterol; it enhances the metabolism of cholesterol in the digestive system and helps to transport it through the circulatory system. In bile, lecithin acts like a soap to dissolve fat for digestion and absorption. Lecithin is a major source of choline, a lipotropic substance. Soy also contains soluble fibre that interferes with the absorption and metabolism of cholesterol and thereby decreases serum cholesterol (Lo et al., 1986). Soy is also a good source of minerals like iron and calcium, which can be deficient in the KD.

Use of spices

We encourage the use of spices from the onset and recent evidence points to several advantages of this.

Turmeric

This bright yellow spice, used in curry powder, is derived from the ground root of turmeric (a relative of ginger) and its main active constituent is curcumin. It has been suggested that curcumin has potential as an adjuvant in epilepsy, both to prevent seizures and to protect seizure-induced memory impairment (Mehla et al., 2010). These authors reported that pretreatment with curcumin ameliorates seizures, oxidative stress and cognitive impairment in pentylenetetrazole (PTZ)-induced kindling in rats.

Cumin seeds

The water extract of *Nigella sativa* L. (black cumin seed) may have anticonvulsant effects in children with refractory seizures. Javad and Hassan (2007) administered an aqueous extract of black seed (40 mg/kg every 8 hours) to 20 children for 4 weeks; the mean frequency of seizures decreased significantly ($P < 0.05$) compared with those who were on placebo.

Saffron

In traditional medicine, saffron has been used as an anticonvulsant remedy. The aqueous and ethanolic extracts of stigmas of *Crocus sativus* have been reported to have anticonvulsant activity in PTZ and MES-induced petit mal and grand mal seizures (Hosseinzadeh and Khosravan, 2002). Agents affecting the PTZ test can inhibit absence seizures. Thus *C. sativus* may have some beneficial effect on this kind of seizure in clinical trials. The extracts showed activity against maximal electroshock seizures, implying that they can improve tonic–clonic seizures (Vida, 1995). The ethanolic extract possesses a sedative effect, which is probably responsible for the anticonvulsant effect (Hosseinzadeh and Khosravan, 2002).

Normalization of lipids

High lipid levels are a frequent side effect in the Western KD. A few of our patients had very high lipid levels and on detailed dietary history we found that they were using saturated fats only (ghee/clarified butter and butter). In India our traditional diet pattern contains different types of fat, namely saturated fatty acids (SFA), monounsaturated fatty acids (MUFA) and polyunsaturated fatty acids (PUFA). Our patients were thus put on a mixed oil KD (MOKD) with a ratio of SFA to MUFA to PUFA of approximately 1 : 1.2 : 1.17 and this normalized lipid levels. This MOKD was achieved by using one meal of saturated fats (ghee/butter), two meals with high MUFA (groundnut oil/mustard/olive oil) and one with high PUFA (sunflower/safflower/soyabean/corn oil). The results (Table 24.1) show that our MOKD maintains normal lipid levels independent of calories, ratio used and age of patient.

Despite this advice, a few patients took more SFA and when their lipids were checked it was found that the levels were high. They were then asked to strictly adhere to the advised mixture of fats. Those with very high lipid levels (serum cholesterol levels above 200 mg/dL; serum triglyceride levels above 170 mg/dL) were instructed to use three parts MUFA and 1 part PUFA and no SFA. Other sources of saturated fats like cream and egg yolk were restricted in their diet until lipid levels came down to normal. This shows that restriction of SFA normalizes blood lipids.

Maintaining uric acid in the normal range

The KD as used in most centres does cause a rise in serum uric acid levels in several patients. However, in the Indian KD this problem is not seen. This is probably due to the high proportion of non-vegetarian foods used in the Western KD. High uric acid levels can be reversed by replacing non-vegetarian protein with soy (Box 24.1).

Use of blood ketones to improve efficacy

After an initial improvement in seizure frequency, some of our patients reached a plateau for several months, despite maintaining a stable urine ketone level of 4+. We decided to do simultaneous urine and blood ketone levels at every monthly clinic visit. Seizure control correlates better with blood β-hydroxybutyrate (BHB) levels than urine ketone levels and is more likely when blood BHB levels are greater than 4 mmol/L (Gilbert et al., 2000). In some patients with stable urine ketone levels of 4+ but suboptimal seizure control, we changed the ketogenic ratio or calories to try to reach a higher blood ketone level (target 4–6 mmol/L). Results of this exercise were gratifying (Table 24.2).

Use of high PUFA to improve efficacy

Despite good blood ketone levels, a subset of patients on the KD still did not have adequate seizure control so we looked at whether changing the type of ingested fat would improve the outcome. The MOKD that we use comprises 32.2% PUFA.

Table 24.1 Plasma lipid levels at baseline, 6, 12 and 24 months in patients receiving saturated fat or mixed oil ketogenic diets.

	Saturated fat ketogenic diet (mean level)			Mixed oil ketogenic diet (MOKD) (mean level)			
	Baseline (N=9)	6 months (N=7)	1 year (N=5)	Baseline (N=71)	6 months (N=53)	1 year (N=49)	2 years (N=30)
Total cholesterol (mg/dL)	183	341	312	188	95	111	95
Triglycerides (mg/dL)	120	157	162	156	168	168	152
High-density lipoprotein (HDL) (mg/dL)	44	47	47	41	38	41	44
Low-density lipoprotein (LDL) (mg/dL)	115	259	233	97	111	107	103
Very low density lipoprotein VLDL (mg/dL)	24	33	34	17	20	22	19
Total cholesterol:HDL ratio	4.1	6.8	6.7	4.0	4.2	4.3	4.2
LDL:HDL ratio	2.8	4.3	4.9	2.5	2.9	2.8	2.4

Box 24.1   Case report of the benefit of vegetarian meals on uric acid levels

Patient A was using four non-vegetarian (NV) meals (including egg, chicken and fish) out of the five meals a day. In 3 months, the serum uric acid level rose to 10.2 mg/dL. The patient was advised to switch to four vegetarian meals including soy and one NV meal. With this change, uric acid levels were normalized within a month.

Table 24.2   Example of use of blood ketone levels to improve efficacy of KD in one patient.

Date	Calories	Ratio	Urine ketones	Blood ketones (mmol/L)	Seizure frequency (per day)
Diet start	1400	1.3:1	4+	1.3	34
Post 1 month	1400	1.5:1	4+	3.4	26
Post 2 months	1400	1.8:1	4+	4.8	12
Post 3 months	1400	1.8:1	4+	4.5	8

Box 24.2   Case report of improved seizure control after changing from MOKD to PUFA KD

Patient B was on MOKD for 4 years. She maintained a urine ketone level of 3+ to 4+ throughout the diet treatment but never achieved a constant 4+. She had achieved 75% control in seizures and then reached a plateau. After being shifted from MOKD to PUFA KD on the same calories and ketogenic ratio, she started attaining 4+ urine ketone levels throughout the day and became 99% seizure-free. However, her blood ketone level was 4.5–6 mmol/L on both the MOKD and PUFA KD.

We switched to the exclusive use of safflower oil, which has a higher PUFA content of 78.2%. Later, patients were shifted to safflower oil and flaxseed oil in a ratio of 2:1. Of a total of 18 patients, five had 100% seizure control, six had over 90% seizure control, five had over 50% seizure control and two had less than 50% seizure control. This is illustrated for one patient in Box 24.2.

One of the many proposed mechanisms of the KD is the elevation of PUFA, which could be responsible for the increased resistance to seizures in ketotic brain tissue. Changes in PUFA are of particular interest as they have been shown to directly modulate the excitability of neurones (Fraser et al., 2003). Animal studies have demonstrated alterations in serum fatty acid levels on the KD. An increase in circulating BHB was reported in rats consuming a flaxseed oil diet (high in PUFA) compared with animals receiving a diet high in SFA (lard, butter diet) or controlled diet (Likhodii et al., 2000). Fuehrelin et al. (2004) reported that a PUFA-enriched KD was capable of achieving a level of ketosis greater than that from a traditional SFA KD in humans, consistent with results obtained in animals, and suggested that a regimen high in MUFA might be expected to yield results similar to those of the PUFA-enriched KD. Lower fasting blood glucose levels and elevated ketones were seen in rats fed safflower oil (high in PUFA) compared with rats fed saturated fats.

Fraser et al. (2003) reported elevated BHB and cortisol levels in children with epilepsy on a KD. In these children, free fatty acids increased 2.2 fold after starting a KD, with significant elevations in most PUFA (arachidonate increased 1.6–2.9 fold and docosahexanoate increased 1.5–4.0 fold). The rise in arachidonate correlated with improved seizure control. Both arachidonate and docosahexanoate inhibit voltage-gated sodium channels and thereby reduce action potential firing of neurones. Given the similar modes of sodium channel inhibition with both PUFA and clinically relevant anticonvulsants (i.e. phenytoin), it is suggested that PUFA may be the endogenous ligands mimicked by these medications. It is therefore possible that the elevation of PUFA on the KD may represent an underlying key anticonvulsant mechanism.

Use of KD in other neurological conditions

We have used the KD in one child with an inoperable pontine glioma. She has been on her KD since 18 months of age and the glioma has reduced from 5.1×3.5×3.6 cm to 3.4×3.9×2.5 cm. She is very active and goes to school taking part in all activities.

Spreading the use of KD in India

It is imperative in a large country like India that there should be several centres offering the KD. However, due to physician indifference and often incredulity towards the KD there was poor response to our workshops. After 10 years (1996–2006), following several presentations at national level conferences, 21 teams (doctors and dietitians) have been trained. At present, several centres are actively offering the KD: two centres use the modified Atkins diet almost exclusively while others use mainly the KD.

Acknowledgements

S. Nathan, K. Datey, B. Chadha and D. Khedekar (Dr Nathan's 'Sanjeev' Clinic, Mumbai, India).

References

Fuehrelin, B., Rutenberg, M.S., Silver, J.N. et al. (2004) Differential metabolic effects of saturated versus polyunsaturated fats in ketogenic diets. *J Clin Endocrinol Metab* **89**, 1641–1645.

Fraser, D., Whiting, S., Andrew, R.D., MacDonald, E.A. and Musa-Veloso, K. (2003) Elevated polyunsaturated fatty acids in blood serum obtained from children on the ketogenic diet. *Neurology* **60**, 1026–1029.

Gilbert, D.L., Pyzik, P.L. and Freeman, J.M. (2000) The ketogenic diet: seizure control correlates better with serum beta-hydroxybutyrate than with urine ketone levels. *J Child Neurol* **15**, 787–790.

Hosseinzadeh, H. and Khosravan, V.V. (2002) Anticonvulsant effects of aqueous and ethanolic extracts of *Crocus sativus* L. stigmas in mice. *Arch Iran Med* **5**, 44–47.

Javad, A. and Hassan, R. (2007) The effect of *Nigella sativa* L. (black cumin seed) on intractable pediatric seizures. *Medical Science Monitor* **13**, 555–559.

Likhodii, S.S., Musa, K., Mendonca, A., Dell, C., Burnham, W.M. and Cunnane, S.C. (2000) Dietary fat, ketosis and seizure resistance in rats on the ketogenic diet. *Epilepsia* **41**, 1400–1410.

Lo, G.S., Goldberg, A.P., Lim, A., Grundhauser, J.J., Anderson, C. and Schonfeld, G. (1986) Soy fiber improves lipid and carbohydrate metabolism in primary hyperlipidemic subjects. *Atherosclerosis* **62**, 239–248.

Mehla, J., Reeta, K.I., Gupta, P. and Gupta, Y.K. (2010) Protective effect of curcumin against seizures and cognitive impairment in a pentylenetetrazole-kindled epileptic rat model. *Life Sci* **87**, 596–603.

Potter, S.M., Baum, J.A., Teng, H., Stillman, R.J., Shay, N.F. and Erdman, J.W. (1998) Soy protein and isoflavones: their effects on blood lipids and bone density in postmenopausal women. *Am J Clin Nutr* **68**, S1375–S1379.

Vida, J.A. (1995) Anticonvulsants. In: Foye, W.O., Lemke, T.L. and Williams, D.A. (eds) *Principles of Medicinal Chemistry*. London: Williams and Wilkins.

Chapter 25

Ketogenic dietary therapy in East Asia

Hoon-Chul Kang and Heung Dong Kim

Severance Children's Hospital and Yonsei University College of Medicine, Seoul, Korea

Since the resurgence of the ketogenic diet (KD) in the mid-1990s, it has been used worldwide for the treatment of refractory paediatric epilepsy (Freeman et al., 2006). However several factors may have contributed to limited availability of the KD for East Asian patients (Kang and Kim, 2006). The KD is generally thought to be intolerable in East Asian countries where the customary diet contains less fat and more carbohydrate than the traditional Western diet. In addition, many Asian countries lack well-trained dietitians and supporting personnel. The lack of experience of physicians and dietitians could also contribute to a negative attitude towards the KD. Despite these limitations, South Korea, Japan, China, Taiwan, Thailand, the Philippines and Hong Kong reportedly offer the KD, and the widespread use of the KD in South Korea is remarkable given the similar food culture to most other Asian countries (Kang et al., 2005; Kossoff and McGrogan, 2005). In South Korea, Dr Heung Dong Kim introduced the KD for the first time for intractable childhood epilepsy in the 1990s and has made efforts to improve the efficacy, safety and tolerability of the diet therapy (Kang et al., 2005; Kang and Kim, 2006).

In Japan, the diet therapy was introduced earlier in the 1970s, but has been mostly used for patients with glucose transporter type 1 (GLUT1) deficiency rather than for intractable epilepsy. More recently, the KD has been recognized as one of the therapeutic modalities for intractable epilepsy, and Dr Hiroshi Maruyama and Dr Tatusya Fuji published a practical guidebook on the KD for dietitians and parents. However, the diet therapy has not yet become popular in Japan.

In China, which accounts for the largest portion of the world's population, several doctors have actively introduced the KD for children with intractable epilepsy. Dr Jianxiang Liao and Dr Chang Xing-Zhi have already accumulated much experience with the KD. In addition, Dr Kuang-Lin Lim, Dr Ching-Shinang

---

Dietary Treatment of Epilepsy: Practical Implementation of Ketogenic Therapy,
First Edition. Edited by Elizabeth Neal.
© 2012 John Wiley & Sons, Ltd. Published 2012 by John Wiley & Sons, Ltd.

Chi and Dr Chao-Ching Huang in Taiwan, Dr Anannit Visudtibhan in Thailand, Dr Benilda C. Sanchez-Gan in the Philippines and Dr Virginia Wong in Hong Kong have reported their anecdotal experiences of the diet therapy.

The KD is no longer unusual in East Asia, and in this chapter we describe our efforts to achieve a safer and more convenient therapeutic diet for refractory paediatric epilepsy.

Implementation of diet therapy

Summary of the suggested protocol (Kang and Kim, 2006)

The KD is indicated for all children, regardless of age and type of epilepsy or epileptic syndrome, but is contraindicated in those with underlying metabolic diseases such as pyruvate carboxylase deficiency and fatty acid oxidation defects. Brief hospitalization for 3–7 days is usually required. The diet begins without initial fasting or fluid restriction, but with only a gradual increase in calories. A fat to non-fat ratio of 4:1 is recommended initially to achieve good ketosis and better efficacy of the KD, and the ratio is then adjusted to 3:1 or to a modified Atkins diet (MAD) to prevent adverse events or improve tolerability of the diet therapy in infants or older children. A short-term trial of the diet for about 6–12 months is usually considered.

Indicated ages

Clinicians have hesitated to prescribe the KD for infants because hypoglycaemia seems to occur more frequently and a long-term unbalanced diet can potentially cause problems in rapidly maturing children. However, the efficacy of the diet in infants and its lack of significant side effects have been reported by some experts (Nordli et al., 2001; Kossoff et al., 2002; Eun et al., 2006). In South Korea, a liquid formula of ketogenic milk has been developed for infants (Kang et al., 2006; Lee et al., 2010). In adolescents, an unpalatable diet may cause resistance and poor compliance, and a reduced ability to extract ketones from the blood into the brain can offset the effectiveness of the KD (Williamson, 1985). However, the maintenance rate and efficacy of the KD do not differ between adolescents and younger children (Kang et al., 2005), with positive attitudes of doctors and parents toward the KD being the most important factors in maintaining the diet. The more nutritionally balanced MAD may help overcome some of these limitations; a small pilot series showed the MAD to be much more tolerable than the KD and as effective in reducing seizure frequency in adolescents and adults with medically resistant epilepsy (Kang et al., 2007a; Smith et al., 2011).

Indicated etiologies

The KD assuages certain disorders of energy metabolism associated with defects in the use of glucose substrates, such as glucose transporter defects and pyruvate dehydrogenase deficiency (De Vivo et al., 1991; Wexler et al., 1997). On the other hand, the KD may be lethal in patients with an underlying metabolic disease, including pyruvate carboxylase deficiency and fatty acid oxidation defects (De Vivo et al., 1977, 1991). The use of the KD has been avoided for patients with mitochondrial respiratory chain defects as the diet can increase the stress on the respiratory chain and tricarboxylic acid cycle (Nordli and De Vivo, 2001). However, the diet therapy has been recently shown to reduce seizure frequency in part by preventing neuronal dysfunction (by decreasing reactive oxygen species and enhancing energy reserves) and stabilizing synaptic transmission (by enhancing energy reserves) (Bough and Rho, 2007). Clinically, we reported for the first time several patients with mitochondrial respiratory chain complex deficiency whose condition was dramatically improved by the KD, without side effects (Kang et al., 2007b).

Initiating the diet

An initial fasting period has been recommended to control seizures by rapidly inducing ketosis and metabolic adaptation to the ketotic state. A period of fasting also provides an opportunity to screen the child for any severe hypoglycaemic predisposition or underlying metabolic disorder (Freeman et al., 2006). In our patients, metabolic adaptation was satisfactorily induced with an initial stepwise caloric increase for 3 days without fasting; dehydration was also less frequent in patients treated without initial fasting than in those treated with initial fasting (Kim et al., 2004). The period of fasting with fluid restriction is emotionally and physically difficult; in order to improve patient compliance with the unbalanced diet, it is important to know that it is not essential.

Duration of the diet

When considering duration of the diet, one might ask why the KD should be maintained for 2 years when seizures respond well, with an additional year for tapering off? It is possible that this protocol was originally based on data for anticonvulsant drugs and has been determined somewhat arbitrarily. For the treatment of infantile spasms, we can consider the following points. The KD has more potent anticonvulsive effects than anticonvulsants, and it possibly has an antiepileptogenic effect. In infants younger than 3 years old (the most appropriate age for the KD), the central nervous system matures very fast. We hypothesized that chronic ketosis lasting for several months might substantially modify the hyperexcitable brain in humans. Recently, Korean researchers compared the prognoses in short-term (8 months) and long-term (more than 2 years) trials involving patients with refractory infantile spasms (Kang et al., 2011). A short-term trial of the KD showed a similar relapse rate compared with a longer duration of KD treatment, and may also reduce other identified long-term adverse effects. Early tapering off of the KD after 6 months could be considered for patients with infantile spasms who become seizure-free.

Development of a liquid formula of ketogenic milk

Two kinds of powdered formula of ketogenic milk that are liquefied with water have been developed. In South Korea, Drs Heung Dong Kim and Dong Wook Kim made a liquid formula of ketogenic milk, Ketonia (Namyang Dairy Products Co., Ltd; Figure 25.1) (Kang et al., 2006; Lee et al., 2010). This does not need to be mixed with water or other food or to be warmed or boiled as it is a ready-to-drink supplementation that makes it easy to use and consume. It was originally developed to increase the tolerability of the diet therapy and also to be used for neonates and infants. The main raw materials of the formula (about 90% of the total energy) are soybean oil and refined high-quality olive oil comprising 18-carbon long-chain fatty acids such as oleic, linolenic and linoleic acids, as well as whey protein concentrate. Since the formula contains mainly olive oil, the liquid ketogenic milk tastes good and fewer gastrointestinal troubles would be expected compared with the conventional KD, which requires patients to consume a high amount of fat

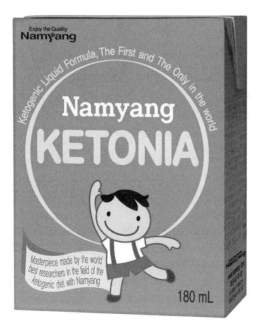

Figure 25.1   A liquid formula of ketogenic milk, Ketonia (Namyang Dairy Products Co., Ltd).

from butter, margarine, mayonnaise, olive and other vegetable oils, and nuts. Moreover, the taste of the formula can be adjusted to resemble that of most other infant formulas or conventional diet.

Development of diverse KD menus

A high amount of fat is the main challenge for the KD and there are limited cooking methods for the KD, such as blending, separating food, stir-frying and deep-frying. Our goal was to develop various recipes and cooking methods to help Korean children adapt to the high-fat diet therapy. We developed five menus: olive oil-based, fish-based, easy-to-cook, for special days, and Ketonia-based (Box 25.1). For each menu, the ratio of fat to carbohydrate plus protein is 4:1 and the total calories are 400 kcal.

Box 25.1   Diverse menus for the KD

Olive oil-based: Keto-summer-roll (Figure 25.2)
- Purpose: to provide a varied and palatable way to consume olive oil.
- Ingredients: chicken, shrimp, sesame leaf, carrot, cucumber, mayonnaise, peanuts, pine nuts and olive oil.
- Recipe: roll chicken, shrimp, cucumber and carrot with a sesame leaf. Make sauce by mixing olive oil, mayonnaise, peanuts, pine nuts and vinegar, salt.
- Feature: it makes it easy to consume olive oil.

Fish-based: Keto-salmon-roll (Figure 25.3)
- Purpose: to combine salmon and vegetables in a palatable menu.
- Ingredients: salmon, cheese, eggplant, cucumber, carrot, milk and olive oil.

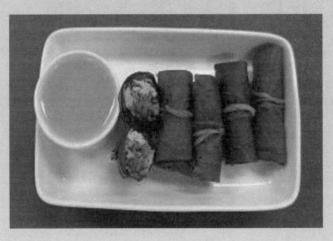

Figure 25.2   Keto-summer-roll.

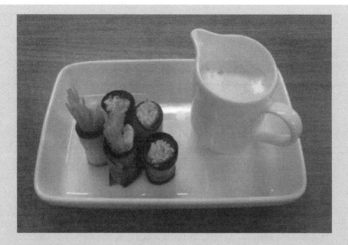

Figure 25.3   Keto-salmon-roll.

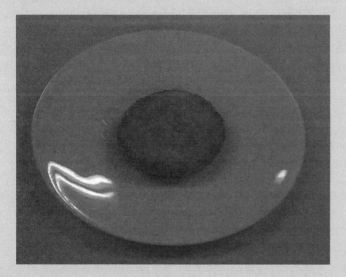

Figure 25.4   Keto-cookie.

- Recipe: roll salmon and carrot with eggplant and cucumber. Blend cheese, milk and olive oil together.
- Feature: it is a good source of the long-chain omega-3 fatty acids, docosahexaenoic acid and eicosapentaenoic acid.

Easy-to-cook: Keto-cookie (Figure 25.4)
- Purpose: to make an easy-to-cook snack.
- Ingredients: egg, whipping cream, butter and olive oil.
- Recipe: blend all ingredients in a mixer. Bake in oven.
- Feature: easy to make. This simple-shaped cookie is popular among our patients.

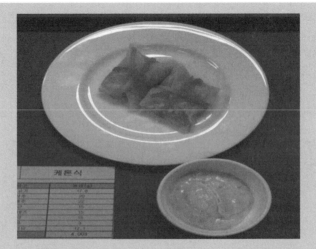

Figure 25.5   Keto-dim sum.

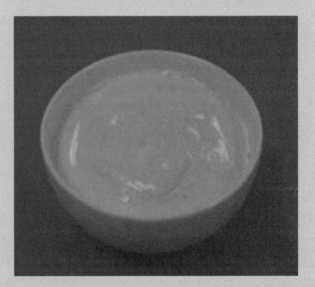

Figure 25.6   Keto-shake.

For special days: Keto-dim sum (Figure 25.5)
- Purpose: to make a menu for special days.
- Ingredients: chicken, cabbage, carrot, mayonnaise, butter, peanuts and olive oil.
- Recipe: stir-fry chopped chicken and carrot. Make a dim sum using cabbage as its skin. Make a dip by mixing olive oil, mayonnaise, butter and chopped peanuts.
- Feature: cabbage is used as dumpling skin.

Ketonia-based: Keto-shake (Figure 25.6)
- Purpose: to provide a varied way to consume Ketonia.
- Ingredients: Ketonia, egg, macadamia nuts, almonds, whipping cream and olive oil.
- Recipe: blend all ingredients in a mixer. Freeze the mix for about 5 hours.
- Feature: paediatric patients prefer this ice cream-like menu.

Modified Atkins diet

The MAD is a more balanced diet compared with the KD (Kossoff et al., 2003). In East Asia, many hospitals have already adopted the MAD as a replacement for the KD for patients who require a long-term trial of the diet therapy and for those who find the KD too restrictive or who develop serious side effects of the KD. A Japanese group of researchers successfully treated a 7-year-old boy with GLUT1 deficiency syndrome with the MAD (Ito et al., 2008). For our patient with Leigh's disease which was caused by a complex IV defect in cytochrome *c* oxidase, the MAD therapy could be helpful (Kim et al., unpublished data).

However, the MAD showed a lower incidence of responders (>50% seizure reduction) than the KD, and it was also more difficult to maintain strong ketosis with the MAD than with the KD (Kang et al., 2007a). Although it is still controversial, maintaining strong ketosis seems to be an important factor in obtaining favourable seizure outcomes from diet therapy. Patients should be more strongly encouraged to consume all diet constituents together and ketosis should be monitored more frequently and carefully when patients are on the MAD compared with the KD.

Concluding remarks

Asian countries have different food cultures, with higher carbohydrate and less fat composition than those of the customary Western diets. Despite this limitation, the KD has been successfully applied as an effective therapeutic modality for intractable childhood epilepsy, thanks to physicians who make continuous efforts to improve the efficacy and tolerability of the diet therapy. In addition to modifying the protocol of the diet therapy, the development of various menus can help children to stay on the unbalanced diet for a long time.

Acknowlegement

We appreciate an excellent dietitian, Eunjoo Lee, for developing a diverse KD menu.

References

Bough, K.J. and Rho, J.M. (2007) Anticonvulsant mechanisms of the ketogenic diet. *Epilepsia* **48**, 43–58.

De Vivo, D.C., Haymond, M.W., Leckie, M.P., Bussman, Y.L., McDougal, D.B. Jr and Pagliara, A.S. (1977) The clinical and biochemical implications of pyruvate carboxylase deficiency. *J Clin Endocrinol Metab* **45**, 1281–1296.

De Vivo, D.C., Trifiletti, R.R., Jacobson, R.I., Ronen, G.M., Behmand, R.A. and Harik, S.I. (1991) Defective glucose transport across the blood–brain barrier as a cause of persistent hypoglycorrhachia, seizures, and developmental delay. *N Engl J Med* **325**, 713–721.

Eun, S.H., Kang, H.C., Kim, D.W. and Kim, H.D. (2006) Ketogenic diet for treatment of infantile spasms. *Brain Dev* **28**, 566–571.

Freeman, J., Veggiotti, P., Lanzi, G., Tagliabue, A. and Perucca, E. (2006) The ketogenic diet: from molecular mechanisms to clinical effects. *Epilepsy Res* **68**, 145–180.

Ito, S., Oguni, H., Ito, Y., Ishigaki, K., Ohinata, J. and Osawa, M. (2008) Modified Atkins diet therapy for a case with glucose transporter type 1 deficiency syndrome. *Brain Dev* **30**, 226–228.

Kang, H.C. and Kim, H.D. (2006) Diet therapy in refractory pediatric epilepsy: increased efficacy and tolerability. *Epileptic Disord* **8**, 309–316.

Kang, H.C., Kim, Y.J., Kim, D.W. and Kim, H.D. (2005) Efficacy and safety of the ketogenic diet for intractable childhood epilepsy: Korean multicentric experience. *Epilepsia* **46**, 272–279.

Kang, H.C., Kim, H.D. and Kim, D.W. (2006) Short-term trial of a liquid ketogenic milk to infants with West syndrome. *Brain Dev* **28**, 67.

Kang, H.C., Lee, H.S., You, S.J., Kang Du, C., Ko, T.S. and Kim H.D. (2007a) Use of a modified Atkins diet in intractable childhood epilepsy. *Epilepsia* **48**, 182–186.

Kang, H.C., Lee, Y.M., Kim, H.D., Lee, J.S. and Slama, A. (2007b) Safe and effective use of the ketogenic diet in children with epilepsy and mitochondrial respiratory chain complex defects. *Epilepsia* **48**, 82–88.

Kang, H.C., Lee, Y.J., Lee, J.S. et al. (2011) Comparison of short- versus long-term ketogenic diet for intractable infantile spasms. *Epilepsia* **52**, 781–787.

Kim, D.W., Kang, H.C., Park, J.C. and Kim, H.D. (2004) Benefits of the nonfasting ketogenic diet compared with the initial fasting ketogenic diet. *Pediatrics* **114**, 1627–1630.

Kossoff, E.H. and McGrogan, J.R. (2005) Worldwide use of the ketogenic diet. *Epilepsia* **46**, 280–289.

Kossoff, E.H., Pyzik, P.L., McGrogan, J.R., Vining, E.P.G. and Freeman, J.M. (2002) Efficacy of the ketogenic diet for infantile spasms. *Pediatrics* **109**, 780–783.

Kossoff, E.H., Krauss, G.L., McGrogan, J.R. and Freeman, J.M. (2003) Efficacy of the Atkins diet as therapy for intractable epilepsy. *Neurology* **61**, 1789–1791.

Lee, Y.J., Kang, H.C., Kim, D.W. et al. (2010) Usefulness of liquid ketogenic milk for intractable childhood epilepsy. *e-SPEN, the European e-Journal of Clinical Nutrition and Metabolism* **5**, e203–e207.

Nordli, D.R. Jr and De Vivo, D.C. (2001) The ketogenic diet. In: Wyllie, E. (ed.) *The Treatment of Epilepsy*, 3rd edn. Philadelphia: Lippincott Williams & Wilkins.

Nordli, D.R. Jr, Kuroda, M.M., Carroll, J. et al. (2001) Experience with the ketogenic diet in infants. *Pediatrics* **108**, 129–133.

Smith, M., Politzer, N., MacGarvie, D., McAndrews, M.P. and Del Campo, M. (2011) Efficacy and tolerability of the Modified Atkins Diet in adults with pharmacoresistant epilepsy: a prospective observational study. *Epilepsia* **52**, 775–780.

Wexler, I.D., Hemalatha, S.G., McConnell, J. et al. (1997) Outcome of pyruvate dehydrogenase deficiency treated with ketogenic diet: studies in patients with identical mutations. *Neurology* **49**, 1655–1661.

Williamson, D.H. (1985) Ketone body metabolism during development. *Fed Proc* **44**, 2342.

Chapter 26

Ketogenic dietary therapy in Africa

Tuscha Du Toit

Specialist Dietitian, Pretoria, South Africa

Background

Of the over 65 million people worldwide who are affected by epilepsy (Ngugi et al., 2010), 80 % are estimated to reside in low- or middle-income countries (World Health Organization, 2005) such as Africa. Dramatic global disparities exist in the availability of care and treatment modalities. The reason for these inequalities may include availability of technologies and reliable drug supply, as well as availability of expertise and access to healthcare (World Health Organization, 2005). Because of the high level of expertise required in selecting suitable candidates, as well as training of health workers, implementation of especially dietary treatments for epilepsy are largely out of reach for many individuals in the developing world. Since no published information is available to indicate how many countries in Africa actually implement the ketogenic diet (KD), it is difficult to give estimates of how many individuals with intractable epilepsy benefit from dietary treatments in this continent. Several referrals from other countries to South Africa suggest that the diet is not implemented in these nations. These include Uganda, Zimbabwe, Namibia, Mozambique and Botswana.

Barriers exist to successful implementation of the KD in Africa. These include, amongst others, limited knowledge, poverty, cultural beliefs, stigma and poor health delivery infrastructure (Mbuba and Newton, 2009; Atadzhanov et al., 2010; Mushi et al., 2011). Despite important advances, a large number of people believe epilepsy to be spiritually rooted, and not medical. Therefore traditional healers play an important and first-priority role compared with medical intervention. In addition, as in the case of Asian countries (Seo and Kim, 2008), carbohydrates, specifically maize flour, are considered to be the main dietary composition of meals in Africa. A huge challenge therefore exists to make the meals culturally acceptable, while still maintaining the efficacy of the diet. However, the main

Dietary Treatment of Epilepsy: Practical Implementation of Ketogenic Therapy,
First Edition. Edited by Elizabeth Neal.
© 2012 John Wiley & Sons, Ltd. Published 2012 by John Wiley & Sons, Ltd.

limitation is probably the small number of dietitians trained and experienced in the implementation of dietary treatments for epilepsy, together with the number and attitude of referring doctors.

In South Africa, KD therapy is not implemented in ketogenic centres at specific hospitals, and no waiting list or evaluation criteria exist to determine who goes onto the diet or not. In the majority of cases, it is implemented with the assistance of a paediatric neurologist and a well-trained experienced dietitian in private practice who specializes in epilepsy. The types of dietary treatment implemented in South Africa include the classical KD, the medium-chain triglyceride (MCT) KD, the modified Atkins diet (MAD) and the low glycaemic index treatment (LGIT) (and in some instances a combination of the treatments).

Food choices

During the assessment consultation the background and diet history of the family is the focus of attention. This information is essential because it indicates the literacy level of the family, whether or not food can be bought, or grown in vegetable gardens, to what degree a variety of food can be included in the diet and whether or not the family would have the money to buy supplements. It would also provide guidance about which one of the dietary treatment choices should be used.

Although KD therapy is not widely used in Africa, it is possible to adapt diets to make the meals culturally acceptable while still maintaining efficacy (Box 26.1). Traditional and typical South African foodstuffs that can be planned as part of a ketogenic meal, especially in the rural areas, include samp and beans, marog (spinach-like vegetable), Orley whip (a protein-free, carbohydrate-free non-dairy cream), atchar (a spicy mango and vegetable mix in an oil base),

---

Box 26.1 Case report illustrating the incorporation of traditional foods into a KD

Patient M was a 9-year-old African boy referred from Uganda. He was diagnosed with Lennox–Gastaut syndrome, and the doctors had very little knowledge regarding the KD. His mother had to save for 2 years to have enough money to come to South Africa, as it was expected that she would stay here for a period of 4–5 weeks. Patient M's seizures were uncontrolled with the anticonvulsant medications lamotrigine and clonazepam and he presented with several myoclonic seizures on a daily basis. He was put on the classical KD at a ratio of 3:1, with 5 mg/kg L-carnitine. He became seizure-free after 3 days. Patient M's family was used to traditional meals, hence the lower ratio to be able to incorporate some of the foodstuffs. A typical meal consisted of

- chicken feet fried in canola oil,
- maas (sour milk) to drink,
- marog and potato, and
- Orley whip.

boerewors (a typical South African sausage), biltong (air-dried beef strips), chicken feet (traditionally boiled or fried in the rural areas), chicken giblets, mopani worms (very high protein source), maas (sour milk), Mahewu (fermented sorghum drink), tinned pilchards and most dried legumes such as kidney beans. It is important to note, however, that these food items are not necessarily representative of our South African culture. Because South Africa is so fortunate to be a 'rainbow nation' with 11 national languages, we have an array of foodstuffs and cultures, most of which are similar to European countries.

Implementation of the KD

In the case of the classical KD, children are not fasted or admitted to hospital during initiation of the diet in order to reduce the costs of hospitalization and to prevent loss of income for parents who have to stay with the children; this is supported by evidence that fasting is not a prerequisite for ketosis and efficacy of the diet (Kim et al., 2004). Prior to starting the diet, the parents are asked to remove all sugars and sweets from the child's habitual diet, and to reduce the carbohydrate portion while increasing the fats. Proper communication is the key to success – almost daily telephone calls and/or email communication provides the support needed. The diet is usually initiated on a lower ketogenic ratio (e.g. 3:1) to accommodate slightly more carbohydrates, and is planned around four meals. To monitor that the children do not become hypoglycaemic or ketoacidotic, each family is given an Abbott Optium Xceed glucometer that can measure both blood glucose and ketone levels, and are then educated on how and when to use it. The glucometer is also used to fine tune the diet in order to reach the most favourable blood glucose and ketone values for optimal seizure control.

Potential triggers for seizure activity are further eliminated from the diet, i.e. caffeine (Ault et al., 1987; Guillet and Dunham, 1995; Zagnoni and Albano, 2002; Kaufman and Sachdeo, 2003) and aspartame. Although we find that optimal seizure control is gained by eliminating aspartame from the diet, scientific evidence is controversial (see Chapter 12). Because of the educational level of several of the patients, a free food exchange system is not implemented in South Africa. In the instances where families do have computers and sufficient literacy levels, they are taught to calculate their own recipes in time, where the dietitian provides the target figures for meal calculations.

With regard to supplementation, a carbohydrate-free vitamin and mineral supplement is given that contains all the 'at-risk' nutrients in sufficient amounts such as calcium, phosphate, selenium and folate, amongst others. Pure L-carnitine is also prescribed as in our experience it may help to prevent, or lower, hypercholesterolaemia. This observation is similar to studies on other groups of patients, not on a KD, that show the lipoprotein-lowering effect of L-carnitine (Sirtori et al., 2000; Derosa et al., 2003). In addition, L-carnitine can help to sustain ketosis (Böhles and Akcetin, 1987). However, it is introduced at a very low dosage (5 mg/kg) and slowly worked up to a concentration of 30–40 mg/kg, as it can induce seizure activity if introduced too quickly. Parents are further urged to focus on polyunsaturated fatty acids when planning recipes to assist in the prevention of hypercholesterolaemia and to supplement with omega-3 fatty acids. Studies show that omega-3 fatty acids increase seizure thresholds and lower inflammatory mediators, which may be increased in people with epilepsy (Schlanger et al., 2002; Taha and McIntyre Burnham, 2007; Yuen et al., 2008).

Modified diets

The MAD and the LGIT are both used in adolescents and adults with intractable epilepsy and may also be implemented in children where compliance is lower. A combination of the two diets is also used, with great efficacy. The LGIT is favoured and easily complied with due to the fact that South Africa places much importance on the glycemic index (GI) in general. The GI Foundation of South Africa (GIFSA) continuously researches, tests and updates typical South African foods to determine their GI value. They further supply books to the consumer with food items listed in colour code (red, high GI; orange, intermediate GI; green, low GI), which increases the understanding of this concept. Our foods are also labelled in such a way as to indicate their GI. In practice, most patients are put on the LGIT, with the understanding that if seizure reduction is not significant, one would move on to the stricter MAD.

References

Atadzhanov, M., Haworth, A., Chomba, E.N., Mbewe, E.K. and Birbeck, G.L. (2010) Epilepsy-associated stigma in Zimbabwe: what factors predict greater felt stigma in a highly stigmatized population? *Epilepsy Behav* **19**, 414–418.

Ault, B., Olney, M.A., Joyner, J.L. et al. (1987) Pro-convulsant actions of theophylline and caffeine in the hippocampus: implications for the management of temporal lobe epilepsy. *Brain Res* **426**, 93–102.

Böhles, H.J. and Akcetin, Z. (1987) Ketogenic effects of low and high levels of carnitine during total parenteral nutrition in the rat. *Am J Clin Nutr* **46**, 47–51.

Derosa, G., Cicero, A.F., Gaddi, A., Mugellini, A., Ciccarelli, L. and Fogari, R. (2003) The effect of L-carnitine on plasma lipoprotein(a) levels in hypercholesterolemic patients with type 2 diabetes mellitus. *Clin Ther* **25**, 1429–1439.

Guillet, R. and Dunham, L. (1995) Neonatal caffeine exposure and seizure susceptibility in rats. *Epilepsia* **36**, 743–749.

Kaufman, K.R. and Sachdeo, R.C. (2003) Caffeinated beverages and decreased seizure control. *Seizure* **12**, 519–521.

Kim, D.W., Kang, H.C., Park, J.C. and Kim, H.D. (2004) Benefits of the non-fasting ketogenic diet compared with the initial fasting ketogenic diet. *Pediatrics* **114**, 1627–1630.

Mbuba, C.K. and Newton, C.R. (2009) Packages of care for epilepsy in low- and middle income countries. *PLoS Med* **6**, e1000162.

Mushi, D., Hunter, E., Mtuya, C., Mshana, G., Aris, E. and Walker, R. (2011) Social-cultural aspects of epilepsy in Kilimanjaro region, Tanzania: knowledge and experience among patients and carers. *Epilepsy Behav* **20**, 338–343.

Ngugi, A.K., Bottomly, C., Kleinschmidt, I., Sander, J.W. and Newton, C.R. (2010) Estimation of the burden of active and life-time epilepsy: a meta-analytic approach. *Epilepsia* **51**, 883–890.

Schlanger, S., Schinitzky, M. and Yam, D. (2002) Diet enriched with omega-3 fatty acids alleviates convulsion symptoms in epilepsy patients. *Epilepsia* **43**, 103–104.

Seo, J.H. and Kim, H.D. (2008) Cultural challenges in using the ketogenic diet in Asian countries. *Epilepsia* **49**, 50–52.

Sirtori, C.R., Calabresi, L., Ferrara, S. et al. (2000) L-carnitine reduces plasma lipoprotein(a) levels in patients with hyper Lp(a). *Nutr Metab Cardiovasc Dis* **10**, 247–251.

Taha, A.Y. and McIntyre Burnham, W. (2007) Commentary on the effects of a ketogenic diet enriched with omega-3 polyunsaturated fatty acids on plasma phospholipid fatty acid profile in children with drug-resistant epilepsy. *Epilepsy Res* **76**, 148–149.

World Health Organization (2005) *Atlas: Epilepsy Care in the World*. Geneva: WHO.

Yuen, A.W., Sander, J.W., Fluegel, D. et al. (2008) Omega-3 fatty acid supplementation in patients with chronic epilepsy: a randomized trial. *Epilepsy Behav* **13**, 712–713.

Zagnoni, P.G. and Albano, C. (2002) Psychostimulants and epilepsy. *Epilepsia* **43**, 28–31.

Chapter 27

Ketogenic dietary therapy in neurometabolic disease

Joerg Klepper

Childrens' Hospital Aschaffenburg, Germany

Ketogenic diet (KD) therapy is mainly used for intractable childhood epilepsy; neurometabolic diseases are rare indications for the diet. Several types of KD therapy have been established and are used for all indications according to age and compliance; currently no appropriate data are available that clarify which KD should be applied in specific conditions. In two diseases of brain energy metabolism, glucose transporter type 1 (GLUT1) deficiency and pyruvate dehydrogenase deficiency (PDHD), the diet is the treatment of choice. It provides ketones as an alternative fuel to the brain. In addition, the diet has been used in several other neurometabolic conditions, but the available data are insufficient to recommend the diet as an established treatment (Kossoff et al., 2009).

Applying the diet in neurometabolic conditions is generally very similar to the KD used in intractable childhood epilepsy. The main differences are the duration and thus potential long-term consequences of the diet in these disorders. In intractable childhood epilepsy, seizure control often remains effective if the KD is discontinued after 2 years. In neurometabolic disorders, the developing brain requires significantly more energy than the mature brain; consequently the KD should be started early and maintained into adolescence. In order to maintain compliance the ketogenic ratio has to be adapted to age: in infants (0–2 years of age) a ketogenic ratio of 3 : 1 is used because higher ratios do not provide sufficient protein for growth. In pre-school and school-age children, 3 : 1 and 4 : 1 ratios are adequate. In older children and adolescents, the modified Atkins diet (MAD) appears to be a very good alternative to a classical KD as it is easier to use, more palatable and thus more acceptable in this age group (Kossoff and Dorward, 2008).

The long duration of the KD in neurometabolic disorders also raises concern about long-term adverse effects such as growth retardation, renal stones and

Dietary Treatment of Epilepsy: Practical Implementation of Ketogenic Therapy,
First Edition. Edited by Elizabeth Neal.

altered blood lipids (Vining, 2008). Currently the available data are insufficient but there is some concern about potential osteoporosis and atherosclerosis resulting from a prolonged KD. As such, patients need to be monitored at regular intervals, supplements must be strictly adhered to, and the neurometabolic disorder requiring a long-term KD should be clearly defined.

The ketogenic diet in GLUT1 deficiency syndrome

GLUT1 deficiency syndrome (GLUT1DS) is a disorder of glucose transport into the brain. As glucose is the primary fuel for brain metabolism, the defect in the glucose transporter GLUT1 results in 'brain energy failure'. Ketones enter the brain via a different transport mechanism and serve as an alternative fuel for the brain, restoring brain energy metabolism (Figure 27.1).

Patients with GLUT1DS develop early-onset epilepsy, global developmental delay and a complex movement disorder. They can be diagnosed by lumbar puncture, which shows low glucose in the cerebrospinal fluid in the setting of normal blood glucose concentrations, or by molecular analysis of the *SLC2A1*

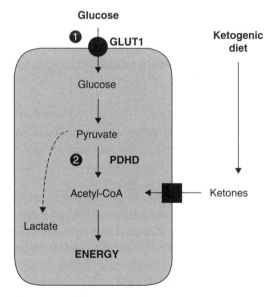

Figure 27.1 Brain energy metabolism, fasting and the ketogenic diet. On a regular diet glucose enters the cell via the GLUT1 glucose transporter (●) and is converted into pyruvate. PDHD converts pyruvate into acetyl-CoA for energy production. Fasting and the ketogenic diet provide ketones that enter the cell via a separate transport system (■) and are metabolized to acetyl-CoA for energy production. Impaired glucose transport into the cell (GLUT1DS, ❶) and pyruvate dehydrogenase deficiency (PDHD, ❷) result in low acetyl-CoA and brain energy failure. Fasting and the ketogenic diet provide ketones as an alternative fuel and restore brain energy production.

gene showing mutations in the gene (Klepper and Leiendecker, 2007; Leen et al., 2010). Recently, several variants of GLUT1DS have been described, including early-onset absence epilepsy, non-epileptic GLUT1DS and paroxysmal exertion-induced dystonia (PED) (Suls et al., 2008; Weber et al., 2008). It is important to diagnose this entity as it represents a treatable childhood epilepsy and the KD currently is the only effective treatment available. In the vast majority of patients, seizures stop with the onset of ketosis; the complex movement disorder and overall development improves remarkably (Klepper et al., 2005).

Except for the duration of the diet, the use of the KD for intractable childhood epilepsy and for GLUT1DS is identical. Ketogenic products, supplements, and dietary control via urinary or blood ketones are the same. However, as there is no alternative to the KD in GLUT1DS, patients and families should be strongly encouraged to maintain the diet. In intractable childhood epilepsy the KD is mostly limited to 2–3 years. In contrast, the diet in GLUT1DS should be started as early as possible and should be maintained throughout childhood as the energy demands of the child's developing brain exceed those of the adult by two to three times, and only return to adult levels in adolescence. In parallel to the general use of the KD, there is increasing evidence that the MAD can offer a good alternative to the classical KD in incompliant patients and teenagers. Currently it remains unclear if there is any benefit in initiating or maintaining the diet in adults with GLUT1DS.

The ketogenic diet in pyruvate dehydrogenase deficiency

PDHD is a severe mitochondrial disorder associated with lactic acidosis, neuro-anatomical defects, developmental delay and early death. Most mutations are located in the X-linked α subunit of the first catalytic component, pyruvate dehydrogenase (E_1). Glucose cannot be metabolized from pyruvate into acetyl-CoA, so pyruvate is metabolized into lactate instead and acetyl-CoA is missing in the respiratory chain for ATP production; thus PDHD resembles another defect of cerebral energy metabolism (Wexler et al., 1997) (Figure 27.1). The early introduction of a KD in PDHD is beneficial based on two mechanisms: (i) the reduction in lactate and pyruvate due to removal of dietary carbohydrate; and (ii) the KD provides ketones as an alternate fuel for the central nervous system and other tissues. Though beneficial, the KD will not completely reverse clinical symptoms (Wexler et al., 1997). In contrast to GLUT1DS, PDHD is a degenerative disease. Often the KD can only delay the progressive loss of abilities and neurological functioning. Also, assessment of the beneficial effects of the KD proves difficult. For instance, some affected children do not have epilepsy; consequently seizure control cannot be applied as a valid parameter. Thus the clinical variability, the neurodegenerative course and the rarity of the disease limit experience and evaluation of the KD in this disorder.

In parallel to GLUT1DS, the practical approach to the KD in PDHD as such does not differ from that in intractable childhood epilepsy. Supplements and a ketogenic ratio of $3:1$ or $4:1$ are required. In severely affected children a permanent gastrointestinal tube for adequate nutrition and hydration may facilitate the application of the KD. To date there is no experience with alternative KD therapies in PDHD and the classical KD is recommended as a lifelong treatment.

The ketogenic diet in other neurometabolic conditions

The successful use of the KD has been reported for several neurometabolic conditions associated with epilepsy (Hartman, 2008; see also Chapter 28). Based on expert opinion, the KD has been beneficial in individual patients but is not currently considered an established treatment for these disorders. Therapeutic mechanisms remain unclear and may be the result of unspecific neuroprotective properties of the KD: ketones provide a more efficient source of energy for brain per unit oxygen and have been shown to decrease cell death in models of Alzheimer and Parkinson disease (Veech et al., 2001). Again, if applied, the KD is in general identical to the KD used for intractable childhood epilepsy.

References

Hartman, A.L. (2008) Does the effectiveness of the ketogenic diet in different epilepsies yield insights into its mechanisms? *Epilepsia* **49** (Suppl. 8), 53–56.

Klepper, J. and Leiendecker, B. (2007) GLUT1 deficiency syndrome: 2007 update. *Dev Med Child Neurol* **49**, 707–716.

Klepper, J., Scheffer, H., Leiendecker, B. et al. (2005) Seizure control and acceptance of the ketogenic diet in GLUT1 deficiency syndrome: a 2- to 5-year follow-up of 15 children enrolled prospectively. *Neuropediatrics* **36**, 302–308.

Kossoff, E.H. and Dorward, J.L. (2008) The modified Atkins diet. *Epilepsia* **49** (Suppl. 8), 37–41.

Kossoff, E.H., Zupec-Kania, B.A., Amark, P.E. et al. (2009) Optimal clinical management of children receiving the ketogenic diet: recommendations of the International Ketogenic Diet Study Group. *Epilepsia* **50**, 304–317.

Leen, W.G., Klepper, J., Verbeek, M.M. et al. (2010) Glucose transporter-1 deficiency syndrome: the expanding clinical and genetic spectrum of a treatable disorder. *Brain* **133**, 655–670.

Suls, A., Dedeken, P., Goffin, K. et al. (2008) Paroxysmal exercise-induced dyskinesia and epilepsy is due to mutations in SLC2A1, encoding the glucose transporter GLUT1. *Brain* **131**, 1831–1844.

Veech, R.L., Chance, B., Kashiwaya, Y., Lardy, H.A. and Cahill, G.F. Jr. (2001) Ketone bodies, potential therapeutic uses. *IUBMB Life* **51**, 241–247.

Vining, E.P. (2008) Long-term health consequences of epilepsy diet treatments. *Epilepsia* **49** (Suppl. 8), 27–29.

Weber, Y.G., Storch, A., Wuttke, T.V. et al. (2008) GLUT1 mutations are a cause of paroxysmal exertion-induced dyskinesias and induce hemolytic anemia by a cation leak. *J Clin Invest* **118**, 2157–2168.

Wexler, I.D., Hemalatha, S.G., McConnell, J. et al. (1997) Outcome of pyruvate dehydrogenase deficiency treated with ketogenic diets. *Neurology* **49**, 1655–1661.

Chapter 28

Beyond epilepsy: ketogenic diet use in other disease states

Adam L. Hartman[1] and Jong M. Rho[2]

[1]Johns Hopkins Hospital, Baltimore, Maryland, USA
[2]University of Calgary Faculty of Medicine and Alberta Children's Hospital, Calgary, Alberta, Canada

That diet and nutrition should influence brain function should not be altogether surprising, but it is only recently that clinicians and investigators have paid close attention to the role that 'metabolic' treatments might play in the treatment of diverse neurological disorders. In the end, a greater mechanistic understanding of neurometabolism in general – from the standpoint of both pathophysiology and identification of targets for therapeutic intervention – will pave the way for novel treatments for a broad spectrum of clinical conditions, but perhaps also for normal brain function throughout the lifespan. This chapter summarizes the rapidly growing literature on how diet may affect a multiplicity of neurological disorders. The reader is referred to other recent sources for more detailed information (Baranano and Hartman, 2008; Maalouf et al., 2009).

Intriguingly, based on the fundamental idea that beneficial metabolic shifts may lead to neuroprotective activity, the ketogenic diet (KD) is increasingly being studied as a potential treatment for a variety of neurological conditions (Box 28.1), both in humans and in animal models (Gasior et al., 2006; Maalouf et al., 2009). While the mechanisms through which the KD exerts such effects are likely diverse, there may indeed be one or more final common pathways that are mechanistically shared. The following briefly summarizes the emerging literature on dietary therapies for neurological diseases, a rapidly expanding area of study.

Alzheimer disease

Alzheimer disease (AD) is characterized by a steady and irreversible decline in cognitive functioning, affecting memory and behaviour, and is associated with a

Dietary Treatment of Epilepsy: Practical Implementation of Ketogenic Therapy,
First Edition. Edited by Elizabeth Neal.

Box 28.1   Neurological conditions potentially treated by a ketogenic diet

Alzheimer disease
Parkinson disease
Amyotrophic lateral sclerosis
Ageing
Ischaemia
Mitochondrial cytopathies
Neurotrauma
Cancer

---

number of abnormalities in metabolism, including toxicity induced by β-amyloid, abnormal glucose control (Sims-Robinson et al., 2010) and glycogen synthase kinase dysfunction (Baum et al., 1996). Thus, it is not surprising that investigators have reasoned the KD might mitigate progression of AD-associated pathology. Class I evidence supporting this hypothesis comes from a randomized, double-blind, clinical, placebo-controlled study of a medium-chain triglyceride (MCT) formulation showing significant improvement in standardized tests of cognitive function in patients with mild-to-moderate AD lacking the APOε4 genotype (Henderson et al., 2009). Interestingly, patients with the APOε4 genotype did not receive similar benefits. At the molecular level, this effect might be mediated by improvements in mitochondrial respiration (Studzinski et al., 2008), evidenced by a protective effect of β-hydroxybutyrate (BHB) on $A\beta_{42}$-induced toxicity in cultured hippocampal neurons (Kashiwaya et al., 2000), or decreased amounts of β-amyloid deposition after treatment with a KD (Van der Auwera et al., 2005). Interestingly, calorie restriction also appears to have a beneficial effect in animal models of AD and this effect may involve SIRT1, a mammalian sirtuin (which, among other actions, deacetylates histones) (Qin et al., 2006; Halagappa et al., 2007). Caution should be exercised in translating these findings to humans, as discrepancies in terms of both clinical efficacy as well as adverse effects have arisen. For example, adverse reactions to calorie restriction have been reported in rodent models (Maalouf et al., 2009).

Parkinson disease

Parkinson disease (PD) is characterized by tremors and difficulty with walking, movement and coordination. The major histopathological feature of PD is the progressive loss of dopaminergic neurons in the substantia nigra pars compacta (SNPC). Improvement in Unified Parkinson Disease Rating Scales (UPDRS) in five adults was noted after treatment with a KD but the possibility that this may have been due to enhanced levodopa absorption has not been ruled out (Vanitallie et al., 2005; Jabre and Bejjani, 2006). Animal data have shown more direct effects. Treatment with BHB protected neurons in the SNPC after administration of 1–methyl-4–phenyl-1,2,3,6–tetrahydropyridine (MPTP), a mitochondrial electron transport chain (ETC) complex I toxin used to model PD (Tieu et al., 2003). This effect may have been mediated by improved mitochondrial oxygen consumption and viability, an effect that appears to require an intact ETC complex II (Tieu et al., 2003). In this context, it is interesting to note that ketone bodies were able to largely prevent ETC complex I and II dysfunction induced by pharmacological inhibitors (Kim do et al., 2010).

Amyotrophic lateral sclerosis

Amyotrophic lateral sclerosis (ALS) is a progressive and fatal motor neuron disease characterized by degeneration of neurons located to the anterior horn of the spinal cord and the cortical neurons that innervate them. A KD led to histological (i.e. motor neuron counts) and functional (time to failure in the Rotarod test) improvements in a transgenic mouse model of ALS (SOD1–G93A) (Zhao et al., 2006). These improvements were thought to be due to increased synthesis rates and concentrations of adenosine triphosphate (ATP), countering the inhibition of complex I of the ETC. A clinical trial is underway to evaluate the effectiveness of a KD in patients with ALS (Clinicaltrials.gov identifier: NCT01035710).

Ageing

The KD has been associated with improvements in an object recognition test and T-maze in aged rats (Xu et al., 2010). In other studies, aged rats were treated with a MCT diet (10 and 20 % MCT) for 8 weeks but changes in synaptic density and synaptic mitochondria were highly dependent on which region was studied (e.g. outer molecular layer of the dentate gyrus vs. stratum moleculare of the CA1 region) (Balietti et al., 2008). The latter suggests more data are needed to evaluate specific effects of the KD on ageing. One particular caveat to note is that such diets – while potentially exerting beneficial effects in multiple disease states – may lead to differential and potentially harmful effects on specific subregions of the brain, particularly during the ageing process (Balietti et al., 2008).

Post-ischaemia models

Prolonged ischaemia leads to activation of metabolic pathways, suggesting that an approach which affects these pathways may mitigate some pathology after these insults (Semenza, 2007). Pretreatment with a KD was associated with decreased hippocampal neurodegeneration and protected cerebellar Purkinje cells and the thalamic reticular nucleus after global cerebral ischaemia in a mouse model (Tai et al., 2008). Pretreatment with either a KD or intracerebroventricular infusion with BHB protected against focal ischaemia as well (Puchowicz et al., 2008). Further, pretreatment with acetoacetate protected against ischaemia in one rat stroke model, as did BHB treatment after the stroke; however, BHB pretreatment was not protective (Massieu et al., 2001; Suzuki et al., 2002). The reason for differences between the two principal ketone bodies is unclear. A KD also may provide benefit in heart muscle after ischaemia, with increased reperfusion recovery in coronary flow, persistence of functional recovery, and increased number of mitochondria compared with rodents fed a regular diet (Al-Zaid et al., 2007).

Mitochondrial cytopathies

Given the importance of mitochondria in metabolism and neuroprotection, a KD might also play a role in treating intrinsic mitochondrial disorders (Bough and Rho, 2007). Patients with disorders of fatty acid oxidation cannot tolerate a KD, but patients with other mitochondrial disorders might benefit from it (Kang et al., 2007). Improvements in mitochondrial architecture have been noted after 'Deletor' mice (who accumulate mitochondrial DNA mutations as they age) were treated with a KD (Ahola-Erkkila et al., 2010), analogous to findings in cultured cells (Santra et al., 2004).

Neurotrauma

A KD prevents cortical contusion volume in juvenile rats in a controlled cortical impact model of traumatic brain injury (Prins et al., 2005). This age-specific protection is associated with decreased utilization of glucose and increased ketone body availability seen with a KD (Prins and Hovda, 2009). Extending these findings in the same model, 24 hours of KD consumption reversed deficits in levels of ATP and creatine and decreased markers of cellular injury (e.g. lactate and *N*-acetylaspartate) in rats injured on postnatal day 35 (Deng-Bryant et al., 2011). Lack of benefit when the injury was induced on postnatal day 70 lends further support to the concept that younger brains adapt more easily to ketone body metabolism than older ones.

Cancer

Perhaps one of the most compelling uses of the KD may be against malignant cancer. Tisdale and Brennan (1983) observed that non-hepatic tumours had much lower levels of acetoacetate-CoA transferase activity than normal tissue, suggesting a 'therapeutic strategy for selective starvation' of tumours. This group later showed that an 80% MCT diet decreased tumour weight in a murine colon adenocarcinoma model, although a long-chain fatty acid (LCFA)-based

KD did not (Tisdale et al., 1987; Tisdale and Brennan, 1988). A 60% MCT diet was used to treat two patients with malignant astrocytomas that were refractory to other therapies, with one patient showing an excellent long-term outcome (Nebeling et al., 1995). An *ad libitum* LCFA-based KD decreased tumour volume of human prostate cancer cells grafted into mice (Freedland et al., 2008). Interestingly, a similar diet did not slow the growth of mouse malignant astrocytomas but a calorie-restricted normal or KD did, with the suggestion that carbohydrate restriction, rather than ketosis, was the critical antineoplastic factor (Seyfried et al., 2003). A hybrid LCFA/MCT KD supplemented with omega-3 fatty acids also slowed tumour progression in a murine gastric adenocarcinoma model (Otto et al., 2008). Thus, the response to various KDs may be tumour dependent and requires further study. Differences in gene expression may shed light on the metabolic vulnerability of different tumours (Stafford et al., 2010).

Conclusion

Clinical applications of metabolism-based therapy appear to be growing rapidly. Thus, there is a present and urgent need to develop modified dietary formulations with improved efficacy and tolerability. The time-honoured KD has and will continue to serve as the cornerstone for validating metabolic therapy as an emerging strategy for neurological disorders.

Acknowledgements

Supported by the National Institutes of Health Clinician-Scientist Award 1K08NS070931 (A.L.H.) and 1RO1NS070261 (J.M.R.).

References

Ahola-Erkkila, S., Carroll, C.J., Peltola-Mjosund, K. et al. (2010) Ketogenic diet slows down mitochondrial myopathy progression in mice. *Hum Mol Genet* **19**, 1974–1984.

Al-Zaid, N.S., Dashti, H.M., Mathew, T.C. and Juggi, J.S. (2007) Low carbohydrate ketogenic diet enhances cardiac tolerance to global ischaemia. *Acta Cardiol* **62**, 381–389.

Balietti, M., Giorgetti, B., Fattoretti, P. et al. (2008) Ketogenic diets cause opposing changes in synaptic morphology in CA1 hippocampus and dentate gyrus of late-adult rats. *Rejuvenation Res* **11**, 631–640.

Baranano, K.W. and Hartman, A.L. (2008) The ketogenic diet: uses in epilepsy and other neurologic illnesses. *Curr Treat Options Neurol* **10**, 410–419.

Baum, L., Hansen, L., Masliah, E. and Saitoh, T. (1996) Glycogen synthase kinase 3 alteration in Alzheimer disease is related to neurofibrillary tangle formation. *Mol Chem Neuropathol* **29**, 253–261.

Bough, K.J. and Rho, J.M. (2007) Anticonvulsant mechanisms of the ketogenic diet. *Epilepsia* **48**, 43–58.

Deng-Bryant, Y., Prins, M.L., Hovda, D.A. and Harris, N.G. (2011) Ketogenic diet prevents alterations in brain metabolism in young but not adult rats after traumatic brain injury. *J Neurotrauma* **28**, 1813–1825.

Freedland, S.J., Mavropoulos, J., Wang, A. et al. (2008) Carbohydrate restriction, prostate cancer growth, and the insulin-like growth factor axis. *Prostate* **68**, 11–19.

Gasior, M., Rogawski, M.A. and Hartman, A.L. (2006) Neuroprotective and disease-modifying effects of the ketogenic diet. *Behav Pharmacol* **17**, 431–439.

Halagappa, V.K., Guo, Z., Pearson, M. et al. (2007) Intermittent fasting and caloric restriction ameliorate age-related behavioral deficits in the triple-transgenic mouse model of Alzheimer's disease. *Neurobiol Dis* **26**, 212–220.

Henderson, S.T., Vogel, J.L., Barr, L.J., Garvin, F., Jones, J.J. and Costantini, L.C. (2009) Study of the ketogenic agent AC-1202 in mild to moderate Alzheimer's disease: a randomized, double-blind, placebo-controlled, multicenter trial. *Nutr Metab (Lond)* **6**, 31.

Jabre, M.G. and Bejjani, B.P. (2006) Treatment of Parkinson disease with diet-induced hyperketonemia: a feasibility study. *Neurology* **66**, 617; author reply 617.

Kang, H.C., Lee, Y.M., Kim, H.D., Lee, J.S. and Slama, A. (2007) Safe and effective use of the ketogenic diet in children with epilepsy and mitochondrial respiratory chain complex defects. *Epilepsia* **48**, 82–88.

Kashiwaya, Y., Takeshima, T., Mori, N., Nakashima, K., Clarke, K. and Veech, R.L. (2000) D-Beta-hydroxybutyrate protects neurons in models of Alzheimer's and Parkinson's disease. *Proc Natl Acad Sci USA* **97**, 5440–5444.

Kim do, Y., Vallejo, J. and Rho, J.M. (2010) Ketones prevent synaptic dysfunction induced by mitochondrial respiratory complex inhibitors. *J Neurochem* **114**, 130–141.

Maalouf, M., Rho, J.M. and Mattson, M.P. (2009) The neuroprotective properties of calorie restriction, the ketogenic diet, and ketone bodies. *Brain Res Rev* **59**, 293–315.

Massieu, L., Del Rio, P. and Montiel, T. (2001) Neurotoxicity of glutamate uptake inhibition in vivo: correlation with succinate dehydrogenase activity and prevention by energy substrates. *Neuroscience* **106**, 669–677.

Nebeling, L.C., Miraldi, F., Shurin, S.B. and Lerner, E. (1995) Effects of a ketogenic diet on tumor metabolism and nutritional status in pediatric oncology patients: two case reports. *J Am Coll Nutr* **14**, 202–208.

Otto, C., Kaemmerer, U., Illert, B. et al. (2008) Growth of human gastric cancer cells in nude mice is delayed by a ketogenic diet supplemented with omega-3 fatty acids and medium-chain triglycerides. *BMC Cancer* **8**, 122.

Prins, M. and Hovda, D. (2009) The effects of age and ketogenic diet on local cerebral metabolic rates of glucose after controlled cortical impact injury in rats. *J Neurotrauma* **26**, 1083–1093.

Prins, M.L., Fujima, L.S. and Hovda, D.A. (2005) Age-dependent reduction of cortical contusion volume by ketones after traumatic brain injury. *J Neurosci Res* **82**, 413–420.

Puchowicz, M.A., Zechel, J.L., Valerio, J. et al. (2008) Neuroprotection in diet-induced ketotic rat brain after focal ischemia. *J Cereb Blood Flow Metab* **28**, 1907–1916.

Qin, W., Yang, T., Ho, L. et al. (2006) Neuronal SIRT1 activation as a novel mechanism underlying the prevention of Alzheimer disease amyloid neuropathology by calorie restriction. *J Biol Chem* **281**, 21745–21754.

Santra, S., Gilkerson, R.W., Davidson, M. and Schon, E.A. (2004) Ketogenic treatment reduces deleted mitochondrial DNAs in cultured human cells. *Ann Neurol* **56**, 662–669.

Semenza, G.L. (2007) Hypoxia-inducible factor 1 (HIF-1) pathway. *Sci STKE* 2007, cm8.

Seyfried, T.N., Sanderson, T.M., El-Abbadi, M.M., McGowan, R. and Mukherjee, P. (2003) Role of glucose and ketone bodies in the metabolic control of experimental brain cancer. *Br J Cancer* **89**, 1375–1382.

Sims-Robinson, C., Kim, B., Rosko, A. and Feldman, E.L. (2010) How does diabetes accelerate Alzheimer disease pathology? *Nat Rev Neurol* **6**, 551–559.

Stafford, P., Abdelwahab, M.G., Kim do, Y., Preul, M.C., Rho, J.M. and Scheck, A.C. (2010) The ketogenic diet reverses gene expression patterns and reduces reactive oxygen species levels when used as an adjuvant therapy for glioma. *Nutr Metab (Lond)* **7**, 74.

Studzinski, C.M., Mackay, W.A., Beckett, T.L. et al. (2008) Induction of ketosis may improve mitochondrial function and decrease steady-state amyloid-beta precursor protein (APP) levels in the aged dog. *Brain Res* **1226**, 209–217.

Suzuki, M., Kitamura, Y., Mori, S. et al. (2002) Beta-hydroxybutyrate, a cerebral function improving agent, protects rat brain against ischemic damage caused by permanent and transient focal cerebral ischemia. *Jpn J Pharmacol* **89**, 36–43.

Tai, K.K., Nguyen, N., Pham, L. and Truong, D.D. (2008) Ketogenic diet prevents cardiac arrest-induced cerebral ischemic neurodegeneration. *J Neural Transm* **115**, 1011–1017.

Tieu, K., Perier, C., Caspersen, C. et al. (2003) D-Beta-hydroxybutyrate rescues mitochondrial respiration and mitigates features of Parkinson disease. *J Clin Invest* **112**, 892–901.

Tisdale, M.J. and Brennan, R.A. (1983) Loss of acetoacetate coenzyme A transferase activity in tumours of peripheral tissues. *Br J Cancer* **47**, 293–297.

Tisdale, M.J. and Brennan, R.A. (1988) A comparison of long-chain triglycerides and medium-chain triglycerides on weight loss and tumour size in a cachexia model. *Br J Cancer* **58**, 580–583.

Tisdale, M.J., Brennan, R.A. and Fearon, K.C. (1987) Reduction of weight loss and tumour size in a cachexia model by a high fat diet. *Br J Cancer* **56**, 39–43.

Van Der Auwera, I., Wera, S., Van Leuven, F. and Henderson, S.T. (2005) A ketogenic diet reduces amyloid beta 40 and 42 in a mouse model of Alzheimer's disease. *Nutr Metab (Lond)* **2**, 28.

Vanitallie, T.B., Nonas, C., Di Rocco, A., Boyar, K., Hyams, K. and Heymsfield, S.B. (2005) Treatment of Parkinson disease with diet-induced hyperketonemia: a feasibility study. *Neurology* **64**, 728–730.

Xu, K., Sun, X., Eroku, B.O., Tsipis, C.P., Puchowicz, M.A. and Lamanna, J.C. (2010) Diet-induced ketosis improves cognitive performance in aged rats. *Adv Exp Med Biol* **662**, 71–75.

Zhao, Z., Lange, D.J., Voustianiouk, A. et al. (2006) A ketogenic diet as a potential novel therapeutic intervention in amyotrophic lateral sclerosis. *BMC Neurosci* **7**, 29.

Afterword

Early in my career I was asked at interview whether dietetics was a science or an art. I replied that it is both, and nowhere is this more apparent than in the implementation of ketogenic dietary therapy. As a dietitian, it is deeply satisfying to use the science of nutrition, biochemistry and physiology to modulate the process of a disease such as epilepsy. On the other hand, skills of artistry are needed to construct a diet acceptable for a particular child, while maintaining nutritional adequacy and growth despite omitting some major food groups. Analytical and judgemental skills are put to the test in monitoring the effects of the dietary treatment and making adjustments to achieve the required levels of a variety of physical and physiological parameters. The very measurable outcomes which can be achieved are clear to patients and carers as well as health service commissioners.

A survey of UK dietitians was conducted in 2007 to see how many patients were currently on ketogenic dietary therapy (Lord and Magrath, 2010). The answer was 152. It was disappointing that numbers had not increased substantially since a previous survey published 10 years earlier (Magrath et al., 2000) despite increasing scientific publications on successful use of this treatment. Fortunately, in the last few years ketogenic dietary therapy has continued to grow in use and become recognized as a routine part of the treatment pathway for children with intractable epilepsy and glucose transporter 1 deficiency. Although National Health Service funding is now more widely available in the UK, we still rely heavily on the support of patient organizations for new post funding, conference organization and counselling support to individual families as they contend with the day-to-day management of the diet.

As our services expand and we gain more experience it has become clear that one size does not fit all. Many patients need not follow a rigid, carefully calculated, ratio-dependent classical ketogenic diet. Most of us now move

Dietary Treatment of Epilepsy: Practical Implementation of Ketogenic Therapy,
First Edition. Edited by Elizabeth Neal.
© 2012 John Wiley & Sons, Ltd. Published 2012 by John Wiley & Sons, Ltd.

between the different dietary approaches: classical, medium-chain triglyceride, modified Atkins and low glycaemic index protocols all contribute to create a diet that is palatable and acceptable for a particular patient and family but still work to achieve the right overall level of ketosis and seizure control.

Our questions have also moved on beyond efficacy and tolerability. We want to establish whether ketones are the best indicator of an optimal dietary prescription. If not, what would be a better measure and how do glucose levels fit in? Do different degrees of ketosis or dietary components have different effects and does this depend on the condition? As epilepsy is a symptom with different causes, is it possible that different dietary approaches are needed for different epilepsies? Should more attention be paid to the type of fat? Do dietary ratios actually matter if satisfactory ketosis is achieved? How can the possible adverse effects of high levels of ketones on growth and bone health be counteracted? Why does the dietary treatment initially seem to help some children who subsequently have deterioration in seizure control? How can we determine in which children the dietary treatment will be helpful so that it is only offered to those who will benefit? There are many questions, but addressing some of these issues will help to refine our clinical practices to ensure best use of limited professional and financial resources.

A further exciting development has been international meetings devoted to ketogenic dietary therapy, providing an opportunity to develop international collaborations and gain useful insights about implementation of diets in India, China, Japan, Korea and many other countries. The increasing use of this dietary therapy in adults opens new clinical and research possibilities, as does the growing body of evidence suggesting that it may have benefits in conditions beyond epilepsy. For a treatment that has been in use over 90 years, the future is still full of potential and hope.

Katherine Lord
*Chair KetoPAG (Ketogenic Diet Professional
Advisory Group of the UK)*

References

Lord, K. and Magrath, G. (2010) Use of the ketogenic diet and dietary practices in the UK. *J Hum Nutr Diet* **23**, 126–132.

Magrath, G., MacDonald, A. and Whitehouse, W. (2000) Dietary practices and use of the ketogenic diet in the UK. *Seizure* **9**, 128–130.

Appendix

Details of dietetic products included in text (with UK address).

Product name	Product type	Manufacturer
Calogen	Long-chain triglyceride fat emulsion	Nutricia*
Caloreen	Glucose polymer powder supplement	Nestlé[†]
FruitiVits	Vitamin, mineral and trace element mixture in powder form	Vitaflo[‡]
Ketocal	Complete 4:1 ratio ketogenic powdered feed	Nutricia*
KetoCal multifibre LQ	Complete vanilla flavoured 4:1 ketogenic ratio liquid feed with added fibre	Nutricia*
Liquigen	Medium-chain triglyceride fat emulsion	Nutricia*
Maxijul	Glucose polymer powder supplement	Nutricia*
Paediatric Seravit	Vitamin, mineral and trace element mixture (powder)	Nutricia*
Phlexy-vits sachets	Vitamin, mineral and trace element mixture in powder form	Nutricia*
Phlexy-vits tablets	Vitamin, mineral and trace element mixture in tablet form	Nutricia*
Protifar	Protein powder supplement	Nutricia*
Pulmocare	High calorie, low carbohydrate liquid feed designed use in adults with chronic obstructive pulmonary disease	Abbott Nutrition**
Resource Optifibre	Soluble dietary fibre powder	Nestlé[†]
Thixo-D Cal Free	Calorie free thickener	Sutherland Health[§]
Vitajoule	Carbohydrate powder supplement	Vitaflo[‡]
Vitapro	Protein powder supplement	Vitaflo[‡]

*Nutricia Advanced Medical Nutrition, White Horse Business Park, Trowbridge, Wiltshire BA14 OXQ, UK.
[†]Nestlé HealthCare Nutrition, St George's House, Croydon, Surrey CR9 1NR, UK.
[‡]Vitaflo International, Suite 1.11, South Harrington Building, 182 Sefton Street, Brunswick Business Park, Liverpool L3 4BQ, UK.
[§]Sutherland Health Group, Unit 1, Rivermead, Pipers Way, Thatcham, Berkshire RG19 4EP, UK.
**Abbott Nutrition, Abbott House, Vanwall Business Park, Vanwall Road, Maidenhead, Berkshire SL6 4XE, UK.

Dietary Treatment of Epilepsy: Practical Implementation of Ketogenic Therapy,
First Edition. Edited by Elizabeth Neal.
© 2012 John Wiley & Sons, Ltd. Published 2012 by John Wiley & Sons, Ltd.

Index

'Note: Page numbers in *italics* refer to Figures; those in **bold** to Tables'

Dietary Treatment of Epilepsy: Practical Implementation of Ketogenic Therapy,
First Edition. Edited by Elizabeth Neal.
© 2012 John Wiley & Sons, Ltd. Published 2012 by John Wiley & Sons, Ltd.

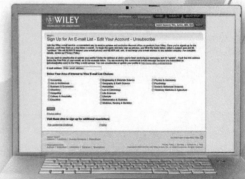
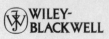